FOGSI EEBR 2025

Ethical Evidence-Based Recommendations

Preterm Labor

Disclaimer

This Ethical Evidence-Based Recommendation (EEBR) document is drafted following a consensus between esteemed FOGSI experts and stakeholders and are based on the scientific evidence available at the time of preparation.

EEBRs should be used for information and educational purposes. They do not replace the need for application of clinical judgment to each individual presentation, or variations based on individual patient and resource setting.

Furthermore, EEBRs do not constitute or imply the endorsement of any of the included technologies, therapies, or techniques by FOGSI.

FOGSI EEBR 2025
Ethical Evidence-Based Recommendations
Preterm Labor

Editor-in-Chief

Sunita Tandulwadkar
MD (Obs and Gyne) FICS (Gyne-Endoscopy) FICOG
President, FOGSI (2025–2026)
Gynecological Endoscopist and ART & IVF Specialist
Head, Department of Obstetrics and Gynecology
Chief, IVF & Endoscopy Center, Ruby Hall Clinic, Pune
Founder and Medical Director
Solo Clinic IVF—A Center for Excellence in Infertility and Endoscopy, Pune
Founder and Medical Director
Solo Stem Cells—A Stem Cell Research and Application Center, Pune
Founder and Director, Alive Regenerative Wellness, Pune, Maharashtra, India

Editor

Laxmi Shrikhande
MBBS MD FRCOG FICOG FICMU FICMCH FIMS
Medical Director and Senior Consultant
Department of Reproductive Medicine
Shrikhande Hospital and Research Centre Pvt Ltd
Nagpur, Maharashtra, India

Experts

Jaideep Malhotra
MBBS MD FIAJAGO FICOG FICMCH FICS FMAS FICMU FRCPI FRCOG FICMP FICRM
Managing Director, ART Rainbow IVF, Agra
Director, Global Rainbow Healthcare, Agra
Director, MHMH (P) Ltd, Agra
President-Elect, In SARG
Past President, FOGSI, ISAR, ASPIRE, IMS, AOGS, SAFOMS, ISPAT
South Asia Director, IAN Donald School
Editor-in-Chief, SAFOG and SAFOMS Journals
Past Vice Chairman, ICOG
Immediate Past Chair, FIGO Committee of Reproductive Endocrinology & Infertility
Past Member, FIGO Working Group on RDEH
Director, SMRITI Manyata CSE
Founder, Club 35 Plus & Rotary Club Agra Grace

Mala Arora
FRCOG (UK) FICOG DA (UK) D Obst (Ire)
Senior Consultant
Department of Obstetrics and Gynecology
Fortis La Femme, New Delhi, India
Founder Director, Indian Recurrent Pregnancy Loss Foundation (IRPL) 2024
Vice President, International Society of Recurrent Pregnancy Loss (ISRPL) 2023
Chairperson, Indian College of Obstetrics & Gynecology (ICOG) 2017
Vice President, FOGSI 2011
Fellow Representative to the RCOG (2007–2017)
Founder President of Faridabad Obstetrics and Gynaecological Society from 2002–2008

Convener

Pooja Lodha
DNB (Obs and Gyne)
Fellow, Fetal Medicine, FOGSI-FMF UK Certified
Lead Consultant
Department of Fetal Medicine
Ruby Hall Clinic and Bharati Vidyapeeth University and Hospital, Pune
Director, Kangaroo Cradle, Fetal Care Centre
Pune, Maharashtra, India

JAYPEE BROTHERS MEDICAL PUBLISHERS
The Health Sciences Publisher
New Delhi | London

Jaypee Brothers Medical Publishers (P) Ltd

Headquarters
Jaypee Brothers Medical Publishers (P) Ltd
EMCA House, 23/23-B
Ansari Road, Daryaganj
New Delhi 110 002, India
Landline: +91-11-23272143, +91-11-23272703
+91-11-23282021, +91-11-23245672
Email: jaypee@jaypeebrothers.com

Corporate Office
Jaypee Brothers Medical Publishers (P) Ltd
4838/24, Ansari Road, Daryaganj
New Delhi 110 002, India
Phone: +91-11-43574357
Fax: +91-11-43574314
Email: jaypee@jaypeebrothers.com

Overseas Office
JP Medical Ltd.
83, Victoria Street, London
SW1H 0HW (UK)
Phone: +44 20 3170 8910
Fax: +44 (0)20 3008 6180
Email: info@jpmedpub.com

Website: www.jaypeebrothers.com
Website: www.jaypeedigital.com

Inquiries for bulk sales may be solicited at: jaypee@jaypeebrothers.com

FOGSI EEBR 2025—Ethical Evidence-Based Recommendations: Preterm Labor

First Edition: **2025**

ISBN: 978-93-6616-876-0

Printed in India

Contributors

Aaishwari Durge
MBBS MS (Obs and Gyne) ICOG
Certification Course in Gynecological
Endoscopy Postgraduate Diploma in ART
and Reproductive Medicine (UKSH-Kiel)
Consultant
Department of Infertility and Gynecology
Oasis Fertility
Hyderabad, Telangana, India

Anumeha Prasad
MD (Obs and Gyne) MRCOG
Senior Clinical Fellow
Department of Obstetrics and Gynecology
Bedford Hospital
Bedfordshire, MK42 9DJ, UK

Apala Priyadarshini
MS (Obs and Gyne)
Assistant Professor
Department of Obstetrics and Gynecology
All India Institute of Medical Sciences
Raebareli, Uttar Pradesh, India

Jaideep Malhotra
MBBS MD FIAJAGO FICOG FICMCH FICS
FMAS FICMU FRCPI FRCOG FICMP FICRM
Managing Director, ART Rainbow IVF, Agra
Director, Global Rainbow Healthcare, Agra
Director, MHMH (P) Ltd, Agra
President-Elect, In SARG
Past President, FOGSI, ISAR, ASPIRE, IMS, AOGS, SAFOMS, ISPAT
South Asia Director, IAN Donald School
Editor-in-Chief, SAFOG and SAFOMS Journals
Past Vice Chairman, ICOG
Immediate Past Chair, FIGO Committee of Reproductive Endocrinology & Infertility
Past Member, FIGO Working Group on RDEH
Director, SMRITI Manyata CSE
Founder, Club 35 Plus & Rotary Club Agra Grace

Laxmi Shrikhande
MBBS MD FRCOG FICOG FICMU FICMCH FIMS
Medical Director and Senior Consultant
Department of Reproductive Medicine
Shrikhande Hospital and Research Centre Pvt Ltd
Nagpur, Maharashtra, India

Mala Arora
FRCOG (UK) FICOG DA (UK) D Obst (Ire)
Senior Consultant
Department of Obstetrics and Gynecology
Fortis La Femme
New Delhi, India
Founder Director, Indian Recurrent Pregnancy Loss Foundation (IRPL) 2024
Vice President, International Society of Recurrent Pregnancy Loss (ISRPL) 2023
Chairperson, Indian College of Obstetrics & Gynecology (ICOG) 2017
Vice President, FOGSI 2011
Fellow Representative to the RCOG (2007–2017)
Founder President of Faridabad Obstetrics and Gynaecological Society from 2002–2008

Mansi Kumar
MD (Obs and Gyne)
Assistant Professor
Department of Obstetrics and Gynecology
Lady Hardinge Medical College and Associated SSK Hospital
New Delhi, India

Ojaswini Patel
MD (Obs and Gyne) FICOG
Professor and Unit Head
Department of Obstetrics and Gynecology
Veer Surendra Sai Institute of Medical Sciences and Research
Sambalpur, Odisha, India

Phalguni Padhi
MD (Ped) DM (Neonatology)
Associate Professor
Department of Neonatology
All India Institute of Medical Sciences
Raipur, Chhattisgarh, India

Pikee Saxena
MD FICOG MNAMS FMAS FIMCH
PGCC (Hospital Management) PGDCR (Clinical Research)
Director–Professor
Department of Obstetrics and Gynecology
Lady Hardinge Medical College and Associated Hospitals
New Delhi, India

Rajshree Katke
MD (Obs and Gyne) FICOG FMAS
Professor and Unit Head
Department Obstetrics and Gynecology
Grant Government Medical College and St George's Hospital
Mumbai, Maharashtra, India

Rekha Rajendrakumar
MD DNB FIRM PGDMLE (Law) FICOG FKCOG FICMCH
Medical Director
Department of IVF and Reproductive Medicine
Chandana Hospital and Miracle IVF
Bengaluru, Karnataka, India
President, Bangalore Society of Obstetrics and Gynecology

Ritu Dargan
MD PGFMLS FICOG FICMCH
Director, Integra Speciality Clinics, Nagpur
Head
Department of Obstetrics and Gynecology
New Era Mother and Child Hospital
Nagpur, Maharashtra, India

Santosh Kumar Dora
MD (Obs and Gyne) Fellowship in Gynecology Oncology
Associate Professor
Department of Obstetrics and Gynecology
Veer Surendra Sai Institute of Medical Sciences and Research
Sambalpur, Odisha, India

Sarita Agrawal
MBBS MD FICOG FIAMS FCGP
Professor and Head
Department of Obstetrics and Gynecology
All India Institute of Medical Sciences
Raipur, Chhattisgarh, India

Shaily Agarwal
MBBS MS FICOG CIMP
Professor and Unit Head
Department of Obstetrics and Gynecology
GSVM Medical College
Kanpur, Uttar Pradesh, India

Shanta Durge
DGO FICOG FKCOG (MRCOG)
Chief Consultant
Department Obstetrics and Gynecology
Durge Clinic and Fertility Centre
Basavakalyan, Karnatak, India
President, Basavakalyan Society of Obstetrics and Gynecology

SP Jaiswar
MS (Obs and Gyne) FICMCH FIAOG FICOG RCOG
Professor and Head
Department of Obstetrics and Gynecology
Era Medical College
Lucknow, Uttar Pradesh, India
President, LOGS (2022–2024)
Editor, Journal of UPCOG
Vice President, UPCOG Chapter

Suchita Tripathi
MBBS MS FMAS DMAS MRCOG
Assistant Professor
Department of Obstetrics and Gynecology
GSVM Medical College
Kanpur, Uttar Pradesh, India

Sudha Sharma
MBBS DGO MD (Community Medicine)
Assistant Professor
Department of Community Medicine
MLB Medical College
Jhansi, Uttar Pradesh, India

Sunita Tandulwadkar
MD (Obs and Gyne) FICS (Gyne-Endoscopy) FICOG
President, FOGSI (2025–2026)
Gynecological Endoscopist and ART & IVF Specialist
Head, Department of Obstetrics and Gynecology
Chief, IVF & Endoscopy Center
Ruby Hall Clinic, Pune
Founder and Medical Director
Solo Clinic IVF—A Center for Excellence in Infertility and Endoscopy, Pune
Founder and Medical Director
Solo Stem Cells—A Stem Cell Research and Application Center, Pune
Founder and Director
Alive Regenerative Wellness
Pune, Maharashtra, India

Urvashi Sharma
MD DNB
Consultant
Department of Obstetrics and Gynecology
New Era Mother and Child Hospital
Nagpur, Maharashtra, India

Vidya Chaudhary
MS (Obs and Gyne) FICOG FCGSM FICMCH
Professor
Department of Obstetrics and Gynecology
Maharani Laxmi Bai Medical College
Jhansi, Uttar Pradesh, India

Preface

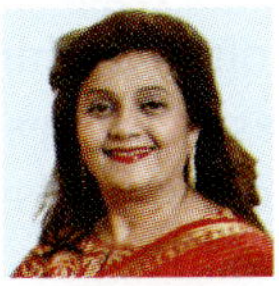

Editor-in-Chief
Sunita Tandulwadkar

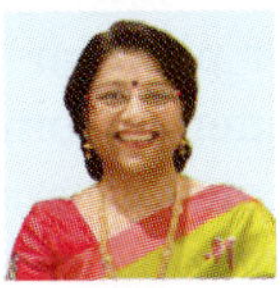

Editor
Laxmi Shrikhande

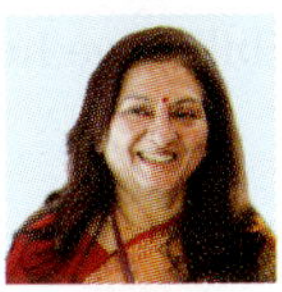

Expert
Jaideep Malhotra

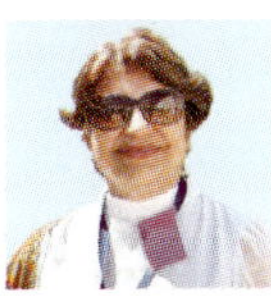

Expert
Mala Arora

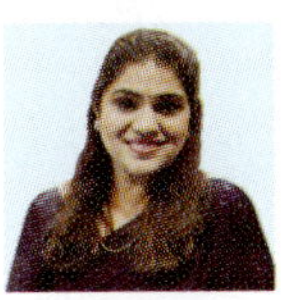

Convener
Pooja Lodha

Preterm labor remains a significant challenge in modern obstetrics, representing a major cause of neonatal morbidity and mortality worldwide. Advances in medicine have undoubtedly expanded our ability to manage preterm births, but the complexity of clinical decision-making in this area demands more than just scientific evidence. It calls for a delicate balance between empirical research, clinical judgment, and ethical considerations. This book, *Ethical Evidence-Based Recommendations on Preterm Labor*, is designed to provide clinicians, researchers, and healthcare policymakers with a comprehensive guide that integrates the latest evidence with the ethical frameworks necessary for informed decision-making.

As healthcare providers, we are often confronted with dilemmas where the best course of action may not always be clear. In the context of preterm labor, where the well-being of both mother and fetus is at stake, our responsibilities are magnified. Every clinical decision, from the administration of tocolytics to the use of antenatal corticosteroids, from fetal monitoring to decisions about neonatal intensive care, carries profound implications. What makes these decisions even more challenging is the need to weigh risks and benefits in situations often characterized by uncertainty. This book aims to empower practitioners with recommendations that are not only rooted in robust evidence but also aligned with ethical principles of beneficence, autonomy, and justice.

The text is structured to guide the reader through the evolving landscape of preterm labor management, beginning with a thorough review of the pathophysiology and risk factors, followed by chapters dedicated to the various interventions available. What distinguishes this work is its emphasis on ethics: Each clinical recommendation is carefully examined through an ethical lens, encouraging reflection on how we, as caregivers, can make compassionate, patient-centered decisions.

In compiling this book, the authors have drawn on a wide array of clinical trials, meta-analyses, and cohort studies to present the most up-to-date and reliable evidence. At the same time, we have consulted ethicists, legal experts, and experienced practitioners to provide insights into the often-ambiguous moral territory that accompanies preterm labor care. The result is a resource that does not simply tell practitioners what to do but rather provides them with the tools to think critically about why and how they should act.

It is our hope that this book will serve as a valuable companion for obstetricians, gynecologists, neonatologists, midwives, and all healthcare professionals involved in the care of women at risk for preterm birth. By integrating evidence with ethics, we strive to promote better outcomes for mothers and their babies while upholding the core values of medical practice.

We are deeply grateful to the numerous experts who contributed to this book and to the patients who have inspired us to keep pushing the boundaries of what is possible in preterm labor care. It is through their courage and resilience that we are reminded of the profound responsibility we hold as healthcare providers.

Contents

CHAPTER 1

Definition, Classification of Preterm Labor

Ritu Dargan, Urvashi Sharma

Q1. How do you define preterm labor?

Ans. The World Health Organization (WHO) has defined preterm labor as the onset of labor after the gestation of viability (20–28 weeks) and before completion of 37 weeks of pregnancy (WHO, 2023).

The American College of Obstetricians and Gynecologists (ACOG) has defined preterm labor as the onset of labor (painful uterine contractions associated with effacement and dilatation of cervix) prior to the completion of 37 weeks (259 days) of gestation counting from the first day of last menstruation period and after the attainment of period of viability (ACOG, 2016).

Q2. How do we classify preterm labor based on gestational age?

Ans. It can be further categorized into early and late preterm. Early preterm is when the baby is born before 33 weeks, and late preterm is when a baby is born between 34 and 36 weeks (Suman and Luther, 2024).

The WHO has classified preterm births as:
- Extremely preterm—those before 28 weeks of gestation.
- Very preterm—those between 28 and 32 weeks of gestation.
- Moderate to late preterm—those between 32 and 37 weeks' gestation.

Q3. What are the signs and symptoms that indicate preterm labor?

Ans. Symptoms of preterm labor include regular contractions before term gestational age associated with cervical change, pelvic pressure, menstrual like cramps, watery vaginal discharge, and lower back pain. Although lower back pain is present in normal pregnancy as well, if occurring before term, it has an established association with impending preterm labor (Suman and Luther, 2024).

If cervical dilatation is noted to be at least 2 or 3 cm at <34 weeks, then the patient is highly likely to deliver preterm. Another indicator is short cervix as assessed by transvaginal ultrasound. Normal cervical length is 35–48 mm. The definition of a short cervix is cervical length <25 mm at 16–24 weeks of gestation.

Q4. How can you diagnose preterm labor definitively?

Ans. Early spontaneous birth can be predicted using serial digital examination or transvaginal ultrasound of the cervix.

Fetal fibronectin detected in cervico-vaginal secretions can also be used.

The diagnosis of true preterm labor that will eventually lead to preterm birth has been facilitated by the use of transvaginal cervical ultrasonography and by the detection of fetal fibronectin in cervicovaginal secretions. The main clinical value of these tests is that preterm birth is very unlikely if the results of both tests are negative. This may help to avoid unnecessary transfer, hospitalization, and treatment of women with false preterm labor (Leitich, 2005).

The detection of phosphorylated insulin-like growth factor binding protein-1 in cervicovaginal secretions, or elevated levels of inflammatory markers, such as interleukin-6, interleukin-8, and tumor necrosis factor-α (TNF-α), also predict preterm birth in symptomatic women. These markers, however, are not routinely used to predict preterm birth in women with symptoms of preterm labor (Leitich, 2005).

BIBLIOGRAPHY

1. American College of Obstetricians and Gynecologists' Committee on Practice Bulletins—Obstetrics. Practice Bulletin No. 171: Management of Preterm Labor. Obstet Gynecol. 2016;128(4):e155-64.
2. Leitich H. Controversies in diagnosis of preterm labour. BJOG: An International Journal of Obstetrics and Gynaecology. 2005;112:61-3.
3. O'Hara S, Zelesco M, Sun Z. Cervical length for predicting preterm birth and a comparison of ultrasonic measurement techniques. Australas J Ultrasound Med. 2013;16(3):124-4.
4. Suman V, Luther EE. Preterm Labor. 2023 Aug 8. In: StatPearls [Internet]. Treasure Island (FL): StatPearls Publishing; 2024 Jan–. PMID: 30725624
5. WHO fact sheet. Preterm birth. [online] Available from https://www.who.int/news-room/fact-sheets/detail/preterm-birth [Last accessed November, 2024].

CHAPTER 2

Pathogenesis, Etiology, and Risk Factors

Shaily Agarwal, Suchita Tripathi

Q1. What are the causes of preterm labor?

Draft recommendations: Preterm labor is now thought to be a syndrome initiated by multiple mechanisms, including infection or inflammation, uteroplacental ischemia or hemorrhage, uterine overdistension, stress, and other immunologically mediated processes however a large population of PTB have no identifiable cause.

The actual etiology of preterm labor is not known, although multiple mechanisms have been propounded for the pathogenesis of preterm labor. For instance, intrauterine infections, inflammation, mechanical stress or overdistension of the uterus, intrauterine growth restriction (IUGR), and uteroplacental hypoxia, or hemorrhage are said to trigger the onset of preterm labor.

Inflammatory response to infection and increased production of matrix metalloproteinases lead to preterm labor. Environmental factors such as exposure to environmental pollutants compromise the immune response to inflammation. Bacterial, viral, and parasitic infections/inflammation such as cervicitis, chronic chorioamnionitis, and deciduitis causes infiltration of the fetal membranes by maternal cytotoxic CD8+T cells, lymphocytes, monocytes, leading to increased gene expression for proinflammatory mediators such as IL-1B, IL-6, TNF-α, and matrix metalloproteinases and resultant preterm labor (Kim CJ et al., 2015). Psychological stress and anxiety increase sympathetic activity and cortisol production with consequent production of corticotropin-releasing hormone leading to preterm labor. Behavioral factors such as smoking and alcohol use cause severe carboxyhemoglobin embryotoxic and teratogenic effects leading to fetal hypoxia, small-for-gestational age, and fetal defects. Nutritional deficiencies lead to premature rupture of the membranes.

Q2. What is the pathophysiology of preterm labor?

Draft recommendations:

- Proinflammatory mediators play a central role in the pathophysiology of preterm labor. Regardless of the stimulus, whether it is mechanical, cytochemical, or hormonal, the final pathway seems to converge toward a central role of inflammatory mediators, i.e., cytokines.

- Increased expression of proinflammatory mediators such as IL-1β, IL-6, IL-8, and TNF-α are associated with increased risk of preterm birth. Available medical therapies for preterm labor have not been consistently effective in aborting uterine contractions during preterm labor due to its ill-defined pathophysiology.

The molecular basis of initiation of labor is unclear but a number of theories for pathophysiology have been proposed. Of these, progesterone withdrawal, oxytocin stimulation, and premature decidual activation are the important ones. Contributory factors such as genetic factors, environmental factors, autoimmune disorders, maternal psychological stress, behavioral factors, e.g., smoking and illicit drugs use, nutritional deficiencies either lead to suppression of immune response to infection which results in activation of inflammatory pathways or they cause increased sympathetic nervous system activity and hypersensitivity to endogenous catecholamines leading to profound vasoconstriction and reduced placental perfusion with resultant restricted fetal growth and birth defects. These pathological mechanisms activate the biological cascade leading to the onset of preterm labor. Whatever the mechanism to initiate labor, three physiological processes have to occur, namely, softening and dilatation of the cervix, uterine myometrial contraction, and weakening and rupture of the membranes.

Proinflammatory mediators play a central role in the pathophysiology of preterm labor and may constitute the main targets for therapeutic interventions in the prevention and clinical management of preterm labor. Imbalances in the pro- and anti-inflammatory pathways may be responsible for preterm labor and post-term pregnancies. Increased expression of proinflammatory mediators such as IL-1β, IL-6, IL-8, and TNF-α, are associated with increased risk of preterm birth. Available therapeutic interventions primarily targeting the proinflammatory pathway seem promising as inflammation plays a central role in the pathogenesis. The basic clinical symptoms of birth canal inflammation are uterine contractions and cervical changes resulting in premature delivery and premature rupture of membranes (PROM).

According to a systemic review (Wei SQ et al., 2010), intrauterine infections is one of the major hypothesized components of inflammatory stimuli which causes increased infiltration of the fetal membranes by white blood cells and plasma cells such as neutrophils, lymphocytes, monocytes, etc. Infiltration of the membranes by these cells is often recognized by pattern recognition receptors such as toll-like receptors found on innate immune cells of the fetal membranes. Activation of these receptors increases gene expression for proinflammatory mediators, including IL-1β, IL-6, IL-8, and TNF-α, while suppressing the expression of IL-4, IL-5, and IL-10 (which place protection role in maintaining uterine quiescence). Proinflammatory mediators cause increased production of prostaglandins (e.g., PGE2,

PGF2), matrix metalloproteinases (MMP-1, -2, -3, etc.) and hyaluronidases. This leads to increased myometrial contractility, preterm premature rupture of the membranes, and cervical ripening and dilation leading to preterm birth.

Q3. What are the risk factors associated with preterm labor?

Draft recommendations:

- Several risk factors for preterm labor are well recognized which includes pre-existing maternal diseases, genetic factors, previous PTB, anatomical factors, and endocrinal factors.
- Other contributing risk factors includes maternal race, ethnicity, age, cigarette smoking, use of ARTs, multifetal pregnancy, etc.

Risk factors for preterm labor:

- Prior preterm birth—Prior preterm birth <34 weeks is among the strongest risk factors
- Poor socioeconomic status
- Low education
- Elderly/teenage pregnancy
- Smoking
- Bleeding in pregnancy
- Assisted reproduction with more than one embryo transfer
- Multiple gestation
- Maternal weight too low or too high
- Concurrent genitourinary tract/periodontal or STI
- Previous surgical MTP
- Uterine anomalies
- Previous cervical surgery
- Short cervix.

According to meta-analysis (Conde-Agudelo et al., 2006), there is a raised risk of preterm birth in pregnancies arising within close temporal proximity to a previous delivery. An interpregnancy interval of <6 months increases >50% risk of preterm birth in present pregnancy. The risk of another preterm birth is inversely related to the gestational age of the previous preterm birth.

Multiple gestations—uterine overdistension, resulting in contractions and PPROM, is believed to be the causative mechanism for the rate of increased spontaneous preterm births.

According to review of literatures (Copper RL et al., 1996, Seldon et al; 1993, RP et al., 2000 and Goldenberg RL et al., 2000), maternal medical disorders, such as thyroid disease, asthma, diabetes, and hypertension, are associated with increased rates of preterm delivery, many of which are indicated because of maternal complications. History of cervical cone biopsy or loop electrocautery excision procedures have also been associated with an increase in spontaneous preterm delivery. Mothers experiencing high levels of psychological or social stress are at increased risk of preterm birth. Women exposed to stressful conditions also have increased serum concentrations of inflammatory markers—such as C reactive protein, an established risk factor for inflammation. According to a review article, smoking is also associated with a systemic inflammatory response and can increase spontaneous preterm birth through inflammatory pathway. Intrauterine infection is a frequent and important mechanism leading to preterm birth.

Research gap: Further research is imperative to uncover the cumulative and specific risk factors associated with PTB. This knowledge is crucial for developing targeted interventions and improving outcomes for at-risk populations.

Q4. What are the predictors of preterm labor?

Draft recommendations: Prediction of preterm labor is difficult due to multiple etiology and lack of enough evidence but there have been attempts to predict preterm labor by considering maternal risk factors including previous obstetric history, maternal infection, ultrasound, and biochemical markers.

The increasing incidence of preterm birth causes a huge economic burden and psychological impact on families and society as the care of preterm babies is highly expensive. Keeping this in mind, the only way to decrease incidence is to predict preterm labor so that timely action can be taken. Prophylactic use of progesterone and cerclage in women with a high risk of preterm birth has been reported to reduce the incidence and improve neonatal outcomes. These results highlight the importance of prediction models in order to establish preventative strategies early in pregnancy.

A single biomarker or even in combination, if found for the prediction of PB can decrease the hospital cost and restrict the treatment and stratification of risk factors is also very important for prevention of preterm birth. Foresight of preterm labor enables taking early action for preterm birth as early referral to higher center, corticosteroids administration, neuroprotective, and antibiotic treatment in case of infection.

Prediction of preterm labor starts with the patient's family history, her socioeconomic status, her educational attainment, age, ethnicity, substance abuse, prior preterm birth, prior surgical intervention, infection in the current pregnancy, multifetal pregnancy, polyhydramnios, etc., among these infections is important causes of preterm birth.

Alteration in vaginal PH from acidic to alkaline in bacterial vaginosis significantly increases the risk of preterm birth and has been considered a significant predictor.

According to a meta-analysis and systemic review (Berghella V et al., 2017 and Son M et al., 2016), screening of cervical length by transvaginal ultrasound is a good predictor of PB risk in singleton pregnancies. The threshold of cervical length in 24 weeks of gestation for PB risk is defined as 25 mm (10th percentile), with 37.3% sensitivity and 92.2% specificity, the knowledge of cervical length had a reduced risk for PB before 37 weeks. A recent study in an extensive population reported that a universal cervical screening program during mid-trimester sonograms in women without a history of preterm birth was associated with a reduction in the PB.

In a comparative study (Banos N et al., 2018), cervical consistency index (CCI), formulated as $(AP^1/AP) \times 100$, measuring anteroposterior cervical diameter before (AP) and after (AP^1) is reported as being more effective than cervical length in prediction of PB.

A systemic review (Honest H et al., 2002), fetal fibronectin is a glycoprotein which is produced by amniocytes and cytotrophoblasts that binds chorionic membranes to maternal decidua. Its presence in cervicovaginal fluid between 24 and 34 weeks of gestation indicates a risk for PB. A systematic review reported that although the accuracy of fetal fibronectin in predicting spontaneous PB varied, it is most accurate in predicting preterm birth in women with threatened preterm labor without advanced cervical dilatation within 7–10 days after testing.

PartoSure a bed side test which measures placental alpha macroglobulin-1 (PAMG-1) shows 80% sensitivity and 95% specificity in prediction of preterm labor and enhance its utility in patients when cervical length was 15–35 mm.

Research gap: More research is required so that preterm labor can be predicted more precisely and timely intervention can be implemented to maximize its benefits.

BIBLIOGRAPHY

1. Banos N, Murillo-Bravo C, Julia C, et al. Mid-trimester sonographic cervical consistency index to predict spontaneous preterm birth in a low-risk population. Ultrasound in Obstet Gynecol. 2018;51(5):629-36.
2. Berghella V, Palacio M, Ness A, et al. Cervical length screening for prevention of preterm birth in singleton pregnancy with threatened preterm labor: systematic review and meta-analysis of randomized controlled trials using individual patient-level data. Ultrasound Obstet Gynecol. 2017;49(3):322-9.
3. Copper RL, Goldenberg RL, Das A. The preterm prediction study: maternal stress is associated with spontaneous preterm birth at less than thirty-five weeks gestation. Am J Obstet Gynecol. 1996;175:1286-92.
4. Goldenberg RL, Hauth JC, Andrews WW. Intrauterine infection and preterm delivery. N Engl J Med. 2000;342:1500-7.

5. Honest H, Bachmann LM, Gupta JK, et al. Accuracy of cervicovaginal fetal fibronectin test in predicting risk of spontaneous preterm birth: systematic review. BMJ. 2002;325(7359):301.
6. Kim CJ, Romero R, Chaemsaithong P, et al. Chronic inflammation of the placenta: definition, classification, pathogenesis, and clinical significance. Am J Obstet Gynecol. 2015;213(4 Suppl):S53-69.
7. Son M, Grobman WA, Ayala NK, et al. A universal mid-trimester transvaginal cervical length screening program and its associated reduced preterm birth rate. Am J Obstet Gynecol. 2016;214(3):365.e1-5.
8. Wei SQ, Fraser W, Luo ZC. Inflammatory cytokines and spontaneous preterm birth in asymptomatic women: A systematic review. Obstet Gynecol. 2010;116(2): 393-401.

CHAPTER 3

Prevention of Preterm Labor

Rekha Rajendrakumar

Q1. How can you prevent preterm labor? How do these methods work to prevent PTL?

Draft recommendations:

- Prior preterm birth is one of the strong predictors of future preterm birth, though there are many other reasons.
- Previous history, frequent monitoring, and assessment of cervical length by TVS in the midterm and use of progesterone and wherever indicated application of cervical cerclage/pessary are the main stay of prevention of preterm labor.

Identifying the risk factors forms the basis of selecting women at risk of preterm labor and needing screening and monitoring for early diagnosis.

- Prior preterm birth—Prior preterm birth <34 weeks is among the strongest risk factors.
- Poor socioeconomic status
- Low education
- Elderly/teenage pregnancy
- Smoking
- Bleeding in pregnancy
- Assisted reproduction with more than one embryo transfer
- Multiple gestation
- Maternal weight too low or too high
- Concurrent genitourinary tract/periodontal or sexually transmitted infections–microorganisms produce endotoxins and phospholipase A2 which cause cell membrane disruption releasing the prostaglandins which in turn induce labor.
- Previous surgical MTP
- Uterine anomalies
- Previous cervical surgery
- Short cervix.

Prevention of preterm labor can be achieved by:

- Since universal screening is not possible, identifying the high risk population, and keeping them under surveillance forms the corner stone of diagnosis and prevention.

- This can be achieved by monitoring the cervical length at the time of NTNB scan between 11 and 13 weeks 6 days (FMF recommendation). The cervical length normally in a primigravida increases till about 20 weeks. The recommendation is at any point of time if the cervical length is <25 mm a cervical cerclage or a pessary should be considered. The other high risk population should be monitored for cervical length serially.
- Prevention, early diagnosis, and early treatment of STI and genitourinary infection
- Treating anemia
- Moderate-to-severe periodontal infections are associated with PTB, attention should be given to oral hygiene.
- Avoid alcohol, illicit substance use, and smoking
- Good nutrition
- Single embryo transfer—PGT-A and single euploid embryo transfer
- Pregnancy spacing
- Altering vaginal microbiome—though this has not been proven to reduce the chances of preterm birth.
- Elective (prophylactic) cervical encerclage—indicated in patients with:
    - history of preterm births
    - classically recurrent and painless second trimester losses
    - funneling of cervix on ultrasound imaging with internal os dilatation of <15 mm
    - short cervix <2.5 cm on TVS examination

Strategies that have no proven efficacy:
- Bed rest
- Hydration
- Avoidance of sexual activity
- Intensive prenatal care
- Empirical use of broad-spectrum antibiotics

Q2. What are the different methods which help to prevent preterm labor?

Draft recommendations:
- Medical management is the first-line of treatment in preventing preterm birth of which progesterone supplementation forms the main cornerstone.
- Some other molecules such as docosahexaenoic acid (DHA) and omega 3 are known to lower the risk of PTB.
- Cervical cerclage/pessary are the interventions which given at the right time in well selected population can prevent PTB.
- *Progesterone:* It is an important molecule in maintenance of the pregnancy and retaining uterine quiescence thus significantly prolonging pregnancy and reducing the numbers of PTB.

- Prophylactic dose of Progesterone—progesterone can be given by various routes and forms namely orally, vaginally, IM, and SC. For long-term use oral and vaginal routes are more compliant than injectables.

Progesterones can be given as:

- *Oral preparations:*
    - Natural micronized progesterone 200–400 mg in divided doses while SR preparations are also available.
    - Dydrogesterone—20–30 mg in divided doses daily.
- *Vaginal preparations:*
    - Vaginal micronized progesterone tablets—200–600 mg per day in divided doses.
    - Progesterone gel 8% 90 mg every night
- *Injectables:*
    - Intramuscular
        - IM progesterone injection 50–100 mg daily
    - Aqueous progesterone injections 25 or 50 mg/day IM or SC.
- Weekly 17 hydroxy progesterone (OHP) injection used earlier is now not recommended as the USFDA approval has been withdrawn because of the possible risks of colorectal, prostate, and brain cancers are higher in pregnancies exposed to it in first trimester and also increase in the incidence of abnormal GTT and GDM.
- Docosahexaenoic acid (DHA)—The KUDOS trial 2016 or the Kansas University DHA Outcome Study (KUDOS) found a significant reduction in the early preterm births with a DHA supplement (which is an omega 3 fatty acid) of 600 mg per day starting from second trimester onward, compared to placebo.
- Cochrane review 2018, which included 70 RCTs involving 19,927 women of mixed population showed high quality evidence that supplementation with 600 mg of omega three long chain poly unsaturated fatty acid (LCPUFA) during the pregnancy lowers the risk of having a preterm baby before 37 weeks by 11%, 34 weeks by 42%, and reduces the risk of having a low-birth-weight baby below 2,500 g by 10%.

Omega 3 has antiprostaglandin action, reduces arachidonic acid reducing the inflammatory action and oxidative stress, thus inhibiting uterine contraction. Maintaining a balance between the metabolites of omega 3 LCPUFA and the proinflammatory omega 6 arachidonic acid is important in maintaining normal gestation length and is a critical element in cervical ripening and the initiation of labor.

Other than increasing gestational length, omega 3 LCPUFA supplements improve child growth and development, preventing childhood allergies, prevention of preeclampsia, decreasing maternal depression, and anxiety.

- Oral probiotics reduce the incidence of vaginal infections, in particular, bacterial vaginosis. Single study is available on this. Evidence is not backed by RCTs.
- *Research gap*—we need more RCTs to know whether oral and/or vaginal probiotics will help to reduce the preterm labor.
- *Cerclage:*
    - Indications
        - History indicated—previous three PTB according to FIGO.
        - USG indicated—TVS cervical length <25 mm at any given time in the second and third trimester.
        - Rescue cerclage—at the time of cervical dilatation.

High order multiple pregnancies have an increased risk of spontaneous PTB yet prophylactic cervical cerclage have not been found to benefit them.

Cervical cerclage is a time tested surgical procedure used globally during pregnancy to reduce the risk of PTB. It can be applied vaginally MacDonald stitch or abdominal Shirodkar stich. Vaginally placed cerclage is lower and considered not as efficacious as abdominal Shirodkar stitch and placement of Shirodkar stitch also involves skill and learning curve. What is universally accepted is that both may play a role in prolongation of pregnancy which ultimately will have reduce the perinatal morbidity and mortality.

Research gap: Prospective studies to assess the characteristics of the procedure and when cervical cerclage will be most beneficial is still lacking.

- Assessment of efficacy of cerclage compared to other treatments in specific groups like previous cervical surgery. Uterine abnormalities, uterine malformations, etc.
- Also need more studies on laparoscopic versus transabdominal stitch.
- Role of adjuvant therapies at the time of cerclage such as antibiotics, tocolytics, and the second suture or a combination of cerclage and pessary.
- Cervical pessary

Research gap: A cervical pessary - Arabin pessary is a silicon ring device that is inserted around the cervix to prevent PTB. Though it is a noninvasive option, its efficiency in comparison to the usual other methods, still needs further evaluation.

Q3. What is the mode of action of progesterone in PTL?

Draft recommendations:

- Progesterone maintains uterine quiescence by many methods, acting at multiple sites.
- Immunomodulation
- Immunomodulation by favoring T2 pathway and tocolysis are the main ways of progesterone action.

Mechanism of action—reduces the risk of preterm birth before 34 weeks thus reducing LBW, perinatal mortality, and NND. Vaginal progesterone decreases preterm birth of <34 weeks of gestation in women with a singleton pregnancy and a short cervix, according to a meta-analysis. In patients at risk of preterm labor, progesterone maintains uterine quiescence by acting at all four sites.

- *At placenta:* Regulates timing of labor via controlling stress hormone.
- *In amniotic fluid:* Limits prostaglandin production.
- *At fetal membranes:* Blocks proinflammatory cytokines induced apoptosis, thus preventing PPROM.
- At myometrium and cervix, suppresses inflammatory response and myometrial contractility.

Other actions of progesterone include:

- Induces secretary transformation of the endometrium that stabilizes and prepares the endometrium for the arriving embryo.
- Promotes local vasodilatation and improves endometrial vascularity.
- Immunomodulation—thus, improves endometrial receptivity.
- Implantation
- Growth of the conceptus
- *Tocolysis:* It inhibits myometrial contractions and maintains uterine quiescence by inducing nitric oxide synthesis in the decidua. Progesterone relaxes myometrial smooth muscle, blocks the action of oxytocin, inhibits the formation of gap junctions and prostaglandin synthesis, and has anti-inflammatory properties, resulting in uterine quiescence.
  Essential immunomodulation is the core property of progesterone.

Beneficial immunomodulation in RPL and preterm labor:

- Th2/Th1 cytokines profile
- Stimulates the production of progesterone induced blocking factor that suppresses natural killer cell activity. This suppressive effect favors implantation and early embryonal development.
- Direct action on NK cell activity—decrease in peripheral NK cell numbers, activation, and cytotoxicity.
- Action on TNF-α and IL-10
- Effect on various protein release
- P makes the embryonic outer trophoblast shell undergo pleomorphism which helps it escape maternal antibody destruction.

Q4. What are the guidelines in prevention of preterm labor?

Draft recommendations:

- Sonographic cervical length measurement should be routinely performed in all pregnant patients once at 11–14 week scan, followed by serial scanning in high risk group.

- Almost all the guidelines endorse that women with a sonographic short cervix (<25 mm) diagnosed in the mid-trimester should be offered daily vaginal micronized progesterone supplementation from second trimester onward up to 36 weeks for the prevention of preterm labor.

  FIGO guideline, 2015 recommends the following:
  - Sonographic cervical length measurement should be performed in all pregnant patients at 19–23 6/7 weeks of gestation using transvaginal ultrasound. This can be done at the same time as the ultrasound performed for the anatomical survey.
  - Women with a sonographic short cervix (<25 mm) diagnosed in the mid-trimester should be offered daily vaginal micronized progesterone supplementation from 19 to 24 weeks up to 36 weeks for the prevention of preterm birth and neonatal morbidity.
  - The progesterone formulation to be used is vaginal micronized progesterone (200 mg vaginal soft capsules) or vaginal micronized progesterone gel (90 mg).
  - Universal cervical length screening and vaginal progesterone treatment (90 mg vaginal gel or 200 mg micronized vaginal soft capsules) is a cost-effective model for the prevention of preterm birth.
- ACOG guidelines—among women with a singleton pregnancy, no history of preterm birth, and cervical length <20 mm at <24 weeks' gestation, vaginal progesterone can reduce the risks for preterm birth and perinatal morbidity and mortality.
- RCOG—progesterone is necessary for successful implantation and the maintenance of pregnancy. This benefit of progesterone could be explained by its immunomodulatory actions in inducing a pregnancy-protective shift from proinflammatory Th-1 cytokine responses to a more favorable anti-inflammatory Th-2 cytokine response.
- WHO—Prenatal administration of progesterone for preventing preterm birth in women considered at risk of preterm birth.
- Society of fetal medicine (SFM) foundation—pregnant women in whom the cervix is prematurely short are at high risk for preterm delivery and should be treated with vaginal progesterone.

BIBLIOGRAPHY

1. Barreto T. Potential of fetal fibronectin testing to prevent preterm birth. Am Fam Physician. 2020;101(11):652-3.
2. Boelig RC, DellaCorte L, Ashoush S, et al. Oral progesterone in prevention of recurrent preterm birth: systematic review and meta-analysis. Am j Obstet Gynecol MFM. 2019;1(1):50-62.
3. Osama El Kady. The value of oral micronized progesterone in the prevention of recurrent spontaneous preterm birth: a randomized controlled trial. Acta Obstet Gynecol Scand. 2017;96:1460-6.

4. Rahman RA, Atan IK, Ali A, et al. Use of the Arabin pessary in women at high risk for preterm birth: long-term experience at a single tertiary centre at Malaysia: BMC Pregnancy and childbirth. 2021;368:21.
5. Solgi E, Tavakoli-Far B, Badehnoosh B, et al. Vaginal and oral probiotics effect in the prevention of preterm delivery in patients visiting Kamali Hospital, Karaj, Iran in 2020. Eur J Obstet Gynecol Reprod Biol. 2022;16:100169.

4

CHAPTER

Management of Preterm Labor

Ojaswini Patel, Santosh Kumar Dora

INTRODUCTION

Preterm birth is a leading cause of perinatal morbidity and mortality worldwide. It is defined as delivery of a newborn prior to 37 completed weeks. The lower cutoff of gestational age varies from country to country mostly 22–24 weeks but ACOG defines the lower cutoff at 20 weeks of gestation.

Category of preterm	*Weeks of delivery*
Extreme preterm	<28 weeks
Very preterm	$28–31^{+6}$ weeks
Moderate preterm	$32–33^{+6}$ weeks
Late preterm	$34–36^{+6}$ weeks

According to WHO, World Association of Perinatal Medicine, Perinatal Medicine Foundation.

There are approximately 15 million preterm births (10% of all deliveries) annually worldwide, of which nearly 80% occurs in Asia and Sub-Saharan Africa. 85% occurs between 32^{+0} to 36^{+6} weeks gestation. 20% of preterm deliveries are contributed by multifocal gestation *(according to WAPM)*

Indian data: Prevalence of preterm labor in India is 23.3% and over 3,500,000 annual preterm births in India.

It can create a broad spectrum of complications ranging from morbidities such as respiratory distress syndrome, intraventricular hemorrhage, necrotizing enterocolitis, bronchopulmonary dysplasia, retinopathy of prematurity, neurodevelopmental problem, and cerebral palsy to perinatal death. Managing preterm labor involves a comprehensive approach aimed at prolonging pregnancy, ensuring fetal well-being, and preparing for potential complications associated with preterm birth. Effective management includes the use of tocolytics, corticosteroids, antibiotics, and sometimes magnesium sulfate for neuroprotection.

Various methods for management of preterm labor are:

- Prevention of preterm labor in high risk mother
- Management of threatened preterm labor
- Management of established preterm labor
- Management of PPROM

RECOMMENDATIONS

- Mothers at increased risk of preterm labor or with signs and symptoms of preterm labor or planned preterm birth should be involved along with the family members and care givers in discussion to make informed choice about their care.
- According to the NICE guideline—information and support to be given as early as possible verbally and in written.
- Information about the likelihood of survival of baby and other outcomes, risk for the babies to be explained.
- Exploration of the neonatal care including the location to be explained.
- Their wishes about resuscitation of the baby to be discussed.

Q1. What is the role of maternal corticosteroids?

Draft recommendations: Corticosteroids are administered to accelerate fetal lung maturity and reduce the risks of respiratory distress syndrome, intraventricular hemorrhage, and neonatal death.

Details—refer corticosteroids section.

Magnesium sulfate for neuroprotection

Magnesium sulfate is used for fetal neuroprotection in women at risk of imminent preterm delivery (before 32 weeks of gestation). It helps reduce the risk of cerebral palsy in preterm infants.

Details—refer magnesium sulfate section.

Q2. What investigations are done while managing preterm labor?

Draft recommendations: Observation of frequency of uterine contractions and demonstrable changes in the cervix as assessed by either a speculum examination or a digital vaginal examination.

Uterine assessment of cervical length is superior to clinical examination.

Fetal fibronectin levels can be used for diagnosis of PTL, wherever available.

Per speculum or digital vaginal examination may not be able to diagnose the early stages of PTL especially dilatation of internal os or cervical funneling thus USG seems to be superior option at that stage.

Though sonographic assessment can be done transvaginal, transabdominal or transperineally; however the transvaginal approach (TVUS) is the gold standard method.

In a meta-analysis of studies in women with symptoms of PTL, using the cervical length (CL) measurement for triage, a CL ≤20 mm or ≤15 mm identified a large proportion of women that delivered within 7 days; overall, only 11% of symptomatic women deliver within 7 days; a CL<15 mm (10% of women) predicted 60% of these cases (90% specificity) and a CL <20 mm predicted 75% of these cases (80% specificity). Importantly, in symptomatic women at <34 weeks, a CL >15 mm had a negative predictive value of 96%, i.e., these women may be reassured that the chance of delivering in the next 7 days is only 4%; also, this negative predictive value did not improve significantly if the cutoff of CL was set at 20 or 25 mm. A more recent Cochrane review examined the effect of the knowledge of CL measurement in singletons with symptoms of PTL. In the knowledge groups, delivery occurred 4 days later (mean difference 0.64 weeks, 95% CI 0.03–1.25; 3 trials, 290 women); however, the results were inconclusive for other outcomes and the evidence was of low-quality (*According to World Association of Perinatal Medicine, Perinatal Medicine Foundation.)*

Biochemical tests: The biochemical markers used in management of threatened PTL include:

- Fetal fibronectin (fFN)—fFN is an extracellular matrix glycoprotein concentrated between the decidua and the trophoblast, found normally in very low levels in cervicovaginal secretions. Levels ≥50 ng/mL between 22 and 34 weeks of gestation have been associated with increased risk of spontaneous preterm birth.
- Phosphorylated Insulin-like growth factor binding protein-1 (phIGFBP-1) is a protein produced by the decidua that may appear in the cervical secretions if uterine contractions disrupt the choriodecidual interface.
- Placental alpha-microglobulin-1 (PAMG) of vaginal fluid is a human protein in the amniotic fluid that is also present in very low levels in the cervicovaginal secretions; cutoff level of 5 ng/mL is usually used to detect preterm labor.

In the prediction of the preterm birth within 7 days in women with signs and symptoms of PTL, the positive predictive value of PAMG-1 was significantly higher than that of PhIGFBP-1 or fFN whereas other diagnostic accuracy measures did not differ. As prevalence affects the predictive performance of a diagnostic test, use of a highly specific assay for a low-prevalence such as PTL may reduce unnecessary treatment significantly (*According to World Association of Perinatal Medicine, Perinatal Medicine Foundation).*

Draft recommendations: FOGSI focus-add year and take it in prediction chapter.

In the patient with history of spontaneous preterm birth/still birth <24 weeks, PPROM, injury to the cervix-serial transvaginal ultrasound for cervical length measurement to be done. Measure TVCL every 14 days from 12 to 24 weeks of gestation, every 7 days, if TVCL<30 mm. If cervical length <25 mm before 24 weeks of gestation cervical cerclage/vaginal progesterone is considered. If there is no high-risk factors TVCL may be measured at 18–24 weeks of gestation and the cutoff limit for prediction of preterm delivery is <25 mm.

World Association of Perinatal Medicine (WAPM): In case of threatened PTL, a stepwise approach should be implemented which includes a period of observation of at least 2 hours, with or without hospital admission. In low resource settings contractions and cervical dilation will guide further management. In high resource settings, further stratification of risk using either ultrasound CL, biomarkers such as fFN or PAMG or a combination of all above should be offered.

NICE Guidelines: Diagnosing of preterm labor for women with intact membranes:

- Clinical history taking
- Observations as per the initial assessment of labor
- Speculum examination (followed by digital examination if required)
- If a swab for fFN is anticipated then it should be taken before any digital vaginal examination.
- If clinical examination suggest that the women is in suspected preterm labor and she is 29^{+0} weeks pregnant or less, advise treatment for preterm labor.
- If clinical examination suggest that the women is in suspected preterm labor and she is 30^{+0} weeks pregnant or more, TVS may be done for cervical length.
    - If CL >15 mm, it is unlikely to be preterm labor.
    - If CL is 15 mm or less, preterm labor is diagnosed and treatment started.
- fFN testing may be done in women who are 30^{+0} weeks pregnant or more if TVS for CL measurement is not available or not acceptable.
- If fFN is negative, it is unlikely, she is in preterm labor.
- If fFN is positive, preterm labor is diagnosed and treatment to be started.
- If women in suspected preterm labor who is 30^{+0} weeks pregnant or more does not have TVS for cervical length or fFN testing, treatment to be offered for preterm labor.
- Do not use TVS for cervical length and fFN testing in combination to diagnose preterm labor.

Q3. What are common tocolytics used in preterm labor?

Ans. Refer to the section of "tocolysis."

Q4. What special precautions for intrapartum management of preterm labor?

Q4A. What is the role of antibiotics and/or probiotics?

Draft recommendations: Antibiotics are administered if preterm labor is associated with premature rupture of membranes (PROM) or if there is evidence of infection.

- *Intrapartum antibiotics:*
    - Once preterm labor is established, antibiotics has no role in preventing labor, but has definite role in treating and preventing infection.
    - The other causes of preterm labor (Like placental insufficiency uterine anomaly, short cervix twins, Polyhydramnios), need to be evaluated properly, and in such cases antibiotics may not have any role.
    - There is lack of evidence regarding the role of probiotics in reduction of PTB however if the PTB is due to the presence of BV , probiotics have been shown to be effective,
- *Guidelines*
    - *ACOG*—screening for bacteriuria in prenatal patients is advised. However, rapid screening tests should not replace urine culture for detecting asymptomatic bacteria. Routine screening for and treatment of asymptomatic BV are not indicated. The use of antibiotics to treat women at high-risk of preterm birth or those with idiopathic spontaneous preterm labor does not significantly decrease the incidence of preterm birth and may result in an increased risk of neonatal developmental abnormalities. This does not preclude the need for prophylaxis against early-onset group B streptococcal disease when indicated. Patients with preterm premature rupture of membranes should receive a 7–10-day course of antibiotic therapy. Antibiotic regimens should include a macrolide (erythromycin or azithromycin) but not ampicillin clavulanic acid *(NICE guideline also supports the use of erythromycin 250 mg 6 hourly for 10 days or till delivery whichever is sooner in case of PPROM).*

Q4B. How should fetal monitoring be done in preterm labor?

Draft recommendations:

- *Regular monitoring of fetal well-being and uterine contractions is essential in managing preterm labor. This includes:*
    - Nonstress tests (NST) and biophysical profiles (BPP) to assess fetal health.
    - Ultrasound to measure cervical length and monitor amniotic fluid levels.

Indications for termination of pregnancy in PTL

- Chorioamnionitis/sepsis
- Fetal distress
- Antepartum hemorrhage requiring immediate delivery
- Preeclampsia/eclampsia requiring delivery
- Abnormal CTG
- Lethal congenital/chromosomal malformation
- Intrauterine fetal death

- Gestational age <24 or >34 weeks
- Maternal comorbidities in which continuation of pregnancy is hazardous
- Advanced cervical dilation
- *Fetal monitoring:* CTG and intermittent auscultation
    - There is limited evidence about usefulness of specific features to suggest hypoxia or acidosis in preterm babies.
    - The available evidence is broadly consistent with that of babies born at term.
    - A normal CTG trace is reassuring but abnormal trace does not necessarily indicate fetal hypoxia or acidosis.
    - *Fetal scalp electrode:* Should not be used below 34 weeks of pregnancy.
    - *Fetal blood sampling:* Should not be used below 34 weeks of pregnancy. It can be used between 34^{+0} and 36^{+6} weeks of pregnancy if benefits outweigh the risk.
- *Mode of birth:*
    - Vaginal birth or CS is done according to the obstetrical situation.
    - No known benefits or harms for the baby from cesarean birth but evidence is very limited.
    - Cesarean birth may be considered between 26^{+0} and 36^{+6} weeks of pregnancy with breech presentation.
- *Timing of the cord clamping:*
    - Wait at least 60 seconds before clamping of the cord unless there is specific maternal or fetal conditions that need earlier clamping.
    - The baby to be positioned at or below the level of placenta before clamping the cord.
- *Special precautions during cesarean section:* Patient may need classical, J-shaped, T-shaped uterine incision for delivering the baby.
- Ensure availability of neonatologist/pediatrician and facilities for NICU.

BIBLIOGRAPHY

1. ACOG Practice Bulletin Clinical Management Guidelines for Obstetrician-Gynecologists Number 217. [online] Available from https://www.acog.org/clinical/clinical-guidance/practice-bulletin [Last accessed November, 2024].
2. Dagklis T, Akolekar R,·Villalain C, et al. Management of preterm labour: Clinical Practice Guideline and Recommendation by the WAPM-World Association of Perinatal Medicine and the PMF-Perinatal Medicine Foundation. EJOG. 2023;291:p196-205.
3. FOGSI. (2017). Focus on prevention of preterm labor. a. [online] Available from https://www.fogsi.org/fogsi-focus-prevention-of-pre-term-labour-2017/ [Last accessed November, 2024].
4. National Institute for Health and Care Excellence (NICE). (2015). Preterm labour and birth. [online] Available from https://www.nice.org.uk/guidance/ng25 [Last accessed November, 2024].

5. RCOG Green-top guideline No. 1b Tocolysis for women in preterm labour. Published February 2011.
6. Royal College of Obstetricians and Gynaecologists. (2022). Cervical cerclage (Green-top Guideline No. 75). [online] Available from https://www:rcog.org.uk/en/guidelimes-research-services/guidelines/gtg75/ [Last accessed November, 2024].
7. Smaill F: Asymptomatic bacteruria in pregnancy. Best Pract Res Clin Obstet Gynaecol. 2007;21:439-50.
8. Tsatsaris V, Papatsonis D, Goffinet F, et al. Nifedipine versus beta-agonists in the management of preterm labor: a meta-analysis. Obstet and Gynecol. 2005; 105(4):980-9.
9. World Health Organization (WHO). (2022). WHO recommendations for care of the preterm or low-birth-weight infant. [online] Available from https://www.who.int/publications/i/item/9789240058262 [Last accessed November, 2024].

CHAPTER 5

Magnesium Sulfate—Roles and Recommendations

Pikee Saxena, Mansi Kumar

INTRODUCTION

Magnesium sulfate is widely used in obstetric care, particularly in the management of preterm pregnancies. Its primary indications include neuroprotection for the preterm fetus and as a tocolytic agent to delay preterm labor.

Q1. What is the role of magnesium sulfate in preterm labor?

Draft recommendations:

- The neuroprotective role for antenatal magnesium sulfate therapy is well established. The exact mechanism of action for magnesium sulfate is unknown; however, there is reduction of vascular instability, preventing hypoxic damage, and mitigating cytokine or excitatory amino acid damage that threaten vulnerable preterm birth.
- Magnesium sulfate is ineffective at delaying birth or preventing preterm birth and its role as tocolytic is questionable, also has no apparent advantages for a range of neonatal and maternal outcomes.

Q2. Mechanism of action of magnesium sulfate

Ans. The mechanism for the neuroprotective effects of magnesium sulfate in preterm infants is not well understood. The following mechanisms have been implicated:

- Stabilization of cerebral circulation by stabilizing blood pressure and normalizing cerebral blood flow.
- Prevention of excitatory injury by stabilization of neuronal membranes and blockade of excitatory neurotransmitters, such as glutamate.

Magnesium is an intracellular cation essential for many enzymatic processes and cellular functions. Magnesium sulfate acts as an endogenous calcium channel antagonist at neuronal synapses, thought to prevent excessive activation of N-methyl-D-aspartate (NMDA) receptors by excitatory amino acids, such as glutamate, and by downregulation of proinflammatory pathways. Early intervention is essential in the prevention of the secondary phase of neuronal injury. The immature brain is particularly prone to excitotoxicity, and inflammation has been strongly implicated in the pathogenesis of cerebral palsy.

Q3. What are regimens and dose of magnesium sulfate?

Ans. The dose of $MgSO_4$ differed between studies, with loading doses varying between 4 g and 6 g, and inconsistency in whether a maintenance dose was administered. A meta-analysis concluded that although the beneficial effect of $MgSO_4$ persisted in the studies using lower overall doses, there is currently insufficient evidence to define a minimum effective dose or optimal regimen for administration. Magnesium toxicity is unlikely at the dose recommended below, and serum magnesium monitoring is not routinely recommended.

Draft recommendations: In women at risk of early preterm birth, use magnesium sulfate for neuroprotection of the fetus:

- Intravenously with a 4 g loading dose (administered slowly over 20–30 minutes).
- 1 g per hour maintenance dose via the intravenous route.
- Continue regimen until birth but stop after 24 hours if undelivered.

The results from the systematic review showed that the most commonly used dosage of 4 g bolus continued by 1 g/hour maintenance, did not increase neonatal mortality and other suspected neonatal complication such as neonatal asphyxia, spontaneous intestinal perforation, necrotizing enterocolitis, and feeding intolerance. Current obstetric standard for use in preterm labor indicates administration of intravenous magnesium sulfate with a loading dose of 4–6 g followed by a maintenance infusion of 1 g per hour until delivery.

Guidelines: The SOGC clinical practice guidelines 2011 based on role of magnesium sulfate for neuroprotection concluded that antenatal magnesium sulfate for fetal neuroprotection reduces the risk of "death or CP" [relative risk (RR) 0.85; 95% confidence interval (CI) 0.74–0.98; 4 trials, 4,446 infants], "death or moderate-severe CP" (RR 0.85; 95% CI 0.73–0.99; 3 trials, 4,250 infants), "any CP" (RR 0.71; 95% CI 0.55–0.91; 4, trials, 4,446 infants), "moderate-to-severe CP" (RR 0.60; 95% CI 0.43–0.84; 3 trials, 4,250 infants), and "substantial gross motor dysfunction" (inability to walk without assistance) (RR 0.60; 95% CI 0.43–0.83; 3 trials, 4,287 women) at 2 years of age.

The 2009 Cochrane review included five randomized control trials involving 6,145 babies of antenatal magnesium sulfate in women at risk of preterm delivery. The review concluded that magnesium sulfate substantially reduced the risk of CP (RR 0.68; 95% CI 0.54–0.87). There was also a significant reduction in gross motor function deficit (RR 0.61; 95% CI 0.44–0.85). However, there was no effect on neonatal mortality (RR 1.04; 95% CI 0.92–1.17). The number of women needed to be treated to benefit one baby by avoiding cerebral palsy is 63 (95% confidence interval 43–155).

Given the beneficial effects of magnesium sulfate on substantial gross motor function in early childhood, outcomes later in childhood should be evaluated to determine the presence or absence of later potentially important neurological effects, particularly on motor or cognitive function.

NICE guidelines (Updated 2022): Give a 4 g intravenous bolus of magnesium sulfate over 15 minutes, followed by an intravenous infusion of 1 g per hour until the birth or for 24 hours (whichever is sooner).

For women on magnesium sulfate, monitor for clinical signs of magnesium toxicity at least every 4 hours by recording pulse, blood pressure, respiratory rate, and deep tendon (for example, patellar) reflexes.

If a woman has or develops oliguria or other evidence of renal failure:
- Monitor more frequently for magnesium toxicity
- Reduce or stop the dose of magnesium sulfate (2015, amended 2022)

Magnesium sulfate has been used in some settings as a tocolytic with the aim of preventing preterm birth however it is ineffective at delaying or preventing preterm birth and has no apparent advantages for a range of neonatal and maternal outcomes.

Its tocolytic efficacy has been found to be similar to that of calcium channel blockers and beta mimetics. The side-effect profile of magnesium sulfate when given for tocolysis is greater than that of other tocolytic agents such as the calcium channel blocker and nifedipine.

Q4. What is magnesium and neurological endpoints trial (MagNET)?

Ans. A total of 1,049 women in preterm labor at 25–33 weeks of gestation (165 fetuses) were included in the MagNET. The tocolytic arm, women in active labor were randomly allocated to receive $MgSO_4$ (4 g bolus then 2–3 g/hour maintenance dose) or another tocolytic agent. In the neuroprotection arm, women with cervical dilatation of >4 cm were randomly allocated to receive $MgSO_4$ (4 g bolus only) or 0.9% saline placebo. Its administration was associated with a reduction in the primary outcome of combined death or cerebral palsy (CP) (RR 0.86, 95% CI 0.75–0.99), and also total CP (RR 0.71, 95% CI 0.55–0.91). There was no increase in the risk of death (RR 0.95, 95% CI 0.80–1.13).

Q5. What is Crowther CA Meta-Analyses (2017)?

Ans. This meta-analysis included individual participant data of five RCTs. All 5 trials identified were included, with 5,493 women and 6,131 babies. It was concluded that antenatal magnesium sulfate given prior to preterm birth for fetal neuroprotection prevents CP and reduces the combined risk of fetal/infant death or CP. Benefit is seen regardless of the reason for preterm birth, with similar effects across a range of preterm gestational ages and different treatment regimens. Widespread implementation globally of this relatively inexpensive, easy-to-administer treatment would lead to important health protection for infants born preterm.

Q6. What are various recommendations for magnesium sulfate?

Ans. Recommendations of NICE Guidelines, 2022:

- In women who have PPROM and are in established labour or having planned preterm birth within 24 hours, intravenous magnesium sulphate should be offered between 24-29+6 weeks of gestation.
- For women between 23^{+0} and 23^{+6} weeks of pregnancy who are in established preterm labor or having a planned preterm birth within 24 hours, discuss with the woman (and her family members or carers, as appropriate) the use of intravenous magnesium sulfate for neuroprotection of the baby, in the context of her individual circumstances **(2019)**.
- Offer intravenous magnesium sulfate for neuroprotection of the baby to women between 24^{+0} and 29^{+6} weeks of pregnancy who are:
    - in established preterm labor, **or**
    - having a planned preterm birth within 24 hours **(2015)**
- Consider intravenous magnesium sulfate for neuroprotection of the baby for women between 30^{+0} and 33^{+6} weeks of pregnancy who are:
    - in established preterm labor, ***or***
    - having a planned preterm birth within 24 hours **(2015)**
- Give a 4 g intravenous bolus of magnesium sulfate over 15 minutes, followed by an intravenous infusion of 1 g per hour until the birth or for 24 hours (whichever is sooner) **(2015)**.
- For women on magnesium sulfate, monitor for clinical signs of magnesium toxicity at least every 4 hours by recording pulse, blood pressure, respiratory rate and deep tendon (for example, patellar) reflexes **(2015)**.
- If a woman has or develops oliguria or other evidence of renal failure:
    - monitor more frequently for magnesium toxicity
    - reduce or stop the dose of magnesium sulfate **(2015, amended 2022)**

FIGO good practice recommendations on magnesium sulfate administration for preterm fetal neuroprotection

- In women at risk of early preterm imminent birth, from viability to 30 weeks of gestation, use of $MgSO_4$ for neuroprotection of the fetus is recommended. In women at risk of early preterm imminent birth, <32–34 weeks of gestation, the use of $MgSO_4$ for neuroprotection of the fetus should be considered.
- $MgSO_4$ should be administered when early preterm birth is planned or expected within 24 hours. When birth is planned, $MgSO_4$ should commence as close as possible to 4 hours before birth. If delivery is planned or expected to occur sooner than 4 hours, $MgSO_4$ should be administered, as there is still likely to be an advantage from administration within this time.

- *In women at risk of early preterm birth, use magnesium sulfate for neuroprotection of the fetus:*
  - Intravenously with a 4 g loading dose (administered slowly over 20–30 minutes)
  - 1 g per hour maintenance dose via the intravenous route.
  - Continue regimen until birth, but stop after 24 hours if undelivered.
- Where $MgSO_4$ is administered, monitor women for clinical signs of magnesium toxicity at least every 4 hours by recording pulse, blood pressure, respiratory rate, and deep tendon (for example, patellar) reflexes.
- In women at risk of imminent preterm birth, $MgSO_4$ should be used for neuroprotection of the fetus, regardless of the cause for preterm birth and the number of babies in utero.

Q7. What are side effects of magnesium sulfate?

Magnesium sulfate produces flushing, sweating, and a sensation of warmth due to its peripheral vasodilator effects when infused intravenously. Other reported maternal side effects related to dosage and speed of infusion include nausea, vomiting, headache, palpitations, and rarely, pulmonary edema. Overdose can result in cardiac and neurological adverse events. There is no evidence of any unintended adverse outcomes in the neonate.

More serious adverse effects which indicate hypermagnesemia are:
- Loss of deep tendon reflexes
- Respiratory depression or arrest
- Cardiac arrest

Other adverse effects may include:
- Thirst
- Muscle weakness
- Headache
- Dizziness
- Hypotension
- Bradycardia

Levels of magnesium sulfate at which adverse effects occur are:
- Symptoms $MgSO_4$ levels (mmol/L)
  - *Feeling of warmth, flushing, double vision, slurred speech:* 3.8–5.0
  - *Loss of tendon reflexes:* >5.0
  - *Respiratory depression:* >6.0
  - *Respiratory arrest:* 6.3–7.0
  - *Cardiac arrest:* >12.0

Stop the infusion and seek medical review if:

- Patellar reflexes are absent
- The respiratory rate is <12 per minute
- The diastolic BP drops >15 mm Hg below baseline
- The urine output drops below 100 mL in 4 hours.

Close clinical monitoring every 4 hourly for deep tendon reflexes, respiratory rate, and urine output is necessary to avoid toxicity.

Magnesium levels may be monitored frequently by checking serum levels every 6–8 hours.

- *Normal serum levels:* 0.7–1.0 mmol/L (1.4–2.0 mEq/L)
- *Therapeutic level in preeclampsia/eclampsia:* 2.0–3.5 mmol/L (4–7 mEq/L)
- *Patellar reflexes lost:* 4.0–5.0 mmol/L (8–10 mEq/L)
- *Respiratory depression:* 5.0–7.5 mmol/L (10–15 mEq/L)
- *Respiratory paralysis:* 6.0–7.5 mmol/L (12–15 mEq/L)
- *Cardiac arrest:* 12.5–15.0 mmol/L (25–30 mEq/L)

Research gap: Multicentric, well designed, adequately powered studies are required to compare different dosage schedules for providing neuroprophylaxis to the fetus.

BIBLIOGRAPHY

1. Bachnas MA, Akbar MIA, Dachlan EG, et al. The role of magnesium sulfate (MgSO4) in fetal neuroprotection. J Matern Fetal Neonatal Med. 2021;34(6):966-78.
2. Costantine MM, Weiner SJ, Eunice Kennedy Shriver National Institute of Child Health and Human Development Maternal-Fetal Medicine Units Network. Effects of antenatal exposure to magnesium sulfate on neuroprotection and mortality in preterm infants: a meta-analysis. Obstet Gynecol. 2009;114:354-64.
3. Crowther CA, Middleton PF, Voysey M, et al. Assessing the neuroprotective benefits for babies of antenatal magnesium sulphate: an individual participant data meta-analysis. PLoS Med. 2017;14(10):e1002398
4. Doyle LW, Crowther CA, Middleton P, et al. Magnesium sulfate for women at risk of preterm birth for neuroprotection of the fetus. Cochrane Database of Systematic Reviews. 2009;(1):CD004661.
5. Hicks MA, Tyagi A. Magnesium Sulfate. In: StatPearls [Internet]. Treasure Island (FL): StatPearls Publishing; 2024.
6. Magee L, Sawchuck D, Synnes A, et al.; Magnesium sulphate for fetal neuroprotection consensus committee; maternal fetal medicine committee. Sogc Clinical Practice Guideline. Magnesium sulphate for fetal neuroprotection. J Obstet Gynecol Can. 2011;33(5):516-29.
7. Royal College of Obstetricians and Gynaecologists. Magnesium Sulphate to Prevent Cerebral Palsy following Preterm Birth. Scientific Impact Paper No. 29. London: RCOG; 2011.

8. Shennan A, Suff N, Jacobsson B; on behalf of the FIGO Working Group for Preterm Birth. FIGO good practice recommendations on magnesium sulfate administration for preterm fetal neuroprotection. Int J Gynecol Obstet. 2021; 155:31-3.
9. Shepherd E, Salam RA, Manhas D, et al. Antenatal magnesium sulphate and adverse neonatal outcomes: a systematic review and meta-analysis. PLoS Med. 2019:16(12):e1002988.

CHAPTER 6

Role of Tocolysis in Preterm Labor

SP Jaiswar, Apala Priyadarshini

Q1. Is the use of tocolysis effective in delaying preterm labor and decreasing adverse neonatal outcomes compared to placebo?

Draft recommendations:

- All classes of tocolytic agents are efficacious in delaying preterm birth by 48 hours up to 7 days compared to placebo.
- The effect of tocolytics on cessation of uterine contractions failed to translate into improving neonatal outcomes in most studies.

Tocolytics are therapeutic agents which cause cessation of uterine contractions to delay preterm birth, allowing time for administration of antenatal corticosteroids, magnesium sulfate for neuroprotection, and in utero transfer of the fetus to a higher center with better neonatal intensive care facilities. Tocolysis is not given with the intention of taking the pregnancy to term but to get a window of opportunity to do the relevant steps necessary to optimize fetal outcomes.

Mayer et al. in a very recent review have mentioned that tocolytics have not been approved by the United States Food and Drug Administration (US FDA) for this purpose. However, they are effective in arresting preterm labor and hence can be used as an off label medication for this indication.

Lamont et al. in their review have mentioned that calcium channel blockers, COX inhibitors, oxytocin receptor antagonists, beta mimetics are superior to placebo/no treatment in arresting preterm labor.

Pinson et al. have also mentioned that the use of tocolytic agents is a good temporary measure to arrest uterine contractions for stabilization of the patients, administration of antenatal corticosteroids, and referral for appropriate care.

In a network meta-analysis published by Cochrane which included 122 trials, all six classes of tocolytic agents were analyzed and their effects in comparison to placebo or no tocolytic treatment were studied. All were effective in delaying preterm birth by 48 hours and 7 days nitric oxide donors being the most efficacious followed by calcium channel blockers and oxytocin receptor antagonists.

A systematic review identified 17 trials (2,800 women) comparing tocolysis with no treatment or placebo. Many trials included maintenance treatment if and after contractions stopped. Some trials excluded women with ruptured membranes but they were included in others. The most frequently evaluated agent was ritodrine. Ritodrine has predominantly beta 2-receptor effects, relaxing muscles in the uterus, arterioles, and bronchi. Other tocolytic drugs evaluated in these trials included isoxsuprine, terbutaline, magnesium sulfate, indomethacin, and atosiban. Overall, tocolytics were associated with a reduction in the odds of birth within 24 hours [odds ratio (OR) 0.47; 95% confidence interval (CI) 0.29–0.77], 48 hours (OR 0.57; 95% CI 0.38–0.83) and 7 days (OR 0.60; 95% CI 0.38–0.95). For the beta-agonists indomethacin and atosiban these effects were statistically significant, but not for magnesium sulfate. However, use of any tocolytic drugs was not associated with a statistically significant reduction in births before 30 weeks of gestation (OR 1.33; 95% CI 0.53–3.33), before 32 weeks of gestation (OR 0.81; 95% CI 0.61–1.07) or before 37 weeks of gestation (OR 0.17; 95% CI 0.02–1.62).

Tocolysis was not associated with a clear reduction in perinatal mortality (OR 1.22; 95% CI 0.84–1.78) nor in neonatal morbidity was it related to being born too early, such as respiratory distress syndrome (OR 0.82; 95% CI 0.64–1.07) or intraventricular hemorrhage (OR 0.73; 95% CI 0.46–1.15).

The ACOG also says that the benefits of tocolytic agents do not simultaneously translate into improving neonatal outcomes.

Q2. What are the tocolytic agents available, their dose, route, mechanism of action, and side effects?

Draft recommendations:

- Calcium channel blockers (nifedipine), nitric oxide donors, cyclooxygenase (COX) inhibitors, oxytocin receptor antagonists are the tocolytic agents available.
- Beta-mimetics should be used with caution despite their good efficacy because of severe maternal side effects.
- Nifedipine may be given at a dose of 20 mg stat orally followed by 1 0 mg 6 hourly. The treatment should be continued till administration of corticosteroids or transfer to a better neonatal healthcare facility or for a duration extending up to 3–7 days.
- The various classes of tocolytics have been summarized in the following table (Patel et al.):

Tocolytic agent	*Dose*	*Route*	*Mechanism of action*	*Adverse effects*
Cyclooxygenase inhibitors	Indomethacin 50–100 mg loading dose, followed by 25 mg orally every 4–6 hours for 48 hours	Oral or rectal	Inhibit prostaglandin synthesis, and hence, inhibit myometrial contractions	Platelet dysfunction, nausea, emesis, gastroesophageal reflux, and gastritis Premature closure of the fetal ductus arteriosus

Contd...

Contd...

Tocolytic agent	***Dose***	***Route***	***Mechanism of action***	***Adverse effects***
Beta mimetics	0.25 mg terbutaline is administered every 20–30 minutes, for up to four doses or till contractions subside 2.5–5 mg/min to a maximum of 25 mg/min	Subcutaneously Intravenous infusion	Cause myometrial relaxation by action beta 2 receptors on myometrial smooth muscle	Nausea and vomiting, palpitations, tachycardia, tremor, headaches, dyspnea, and nonspecific chest pain
Calcium channel blockers	Nifedipine 20 mg stat followed by 10 mg 6 hourly till 3–7 days	Oral	Inhibit calcium influx into smooth muscle cells of myometrium	Most common side effects are hypotension-related symptoms (e.g., supine hypotension) and headache nausea, flushing, dizziness
Oxytocin receptor antagonists	Atosiban bolus of 6.75 mg followed by a 300 µg/min infusion for 3 hours, followed by 100 µg/min infusion for up to 45 hours	Intravenous	Compete with oxytocin receptors in the myometrium and the decidua	Hypersensitivity and injection site reactions
Nitric oxide donors	10 mg glyceryl trinitrate patch is applied to the abdomen. 20 mg/min	Transdermal Intravenous	Nitric oxide leads to increase in cGMP in smooth muscle cells leads to the activation of myosin light chain kinases, which results in smooth muscle relaxation	Headache, dizziness, nausea, vomiting, flushing, palpitations, maternal hypotension

Contd...

Contd...

Tocolytic agent	***Dose***	***Route***	***Mechanism of action***	***Adverse effects***
Magnesium sulfate	4–6 g bolus administered over 20–30 minutes, followed by a continuous intravenous infusion of 1–2 g/hours	Intravenous	Intracellular calcium antagonist hence inhibits myometrial contractions	Flushing, pulmonary edema, cardiac arrest neonatal lethargy and respiratory distress

The decision about the administration of tocolytics should be a shared one after counseling the patient and the family about the possible adverse effects and the consequences.

Beta-agonists have a high frequency of adverse effects. Nifedipine, atosiban, and the COX inhibitors have fewer types of adverse effects, and they occur less frequently than for beta-agonists but how they compare with each other is unclear *(Grade of recommendation-A).*

Using multiple tocolytic drugs appears to be associated with a higher risk of adverse effects and so should be avoided *(Grade of recommendation-B).*

Common adverse effects when beta-agonists are compared with placebo include palpitations (38% for beta-agonists compared with 4% for placebo), tremor (39% compared with 4%), nausea or vomiting (21% compared with 12%), headache (19% compared with 5%), chest pain (10% compared with 1%) and dyspnea (14% compared with 3%). Women allocated beta-agonists were far more likely to stop treatment because of adverse effects than those allocated placebo (five trials, 1,081 women; RR 11.38; 95% CI 5.21–24.86). Rare but serious and potentially life-threatening adverse effects have been reported following beta-agonist use and there are case reports of a small number of maternal deaths associated with use of these drugs. Pulmonary edema is a well-documented complication, usually associated with aggressive intravenous hydration. A systematic review reported one case of pulmonary edema among 852 women (1/425 beta-agonists compared with 0/427 placebo).

In a recent network meta-analysis by Cochrane it was observed that with beta mimetics there is a higher incidence of dyspnea, vomiting, palpitations, headache, and tachycardia as compared to no treatment or placebo treatment. Use of COX inhibitors resulted in more vomiting and calcium channel blockers showed higher incidence of headache as compared to placebo.

Hanley et al. in their review have described in detail the various classes of tocolytics available and have also mentioned that calcium channel blockers were the tocolytics of choice by various healthcare practitioners.

Q3. Which tocolytic should be preferred considering comparative safety and efficacy?

Draft recommendations:

- Nifedipine appeared to be the preferred drug for both acute and maintenance tocolytic therapy in women who were at risk for preterm labor.
- Nitric oxide donors and oxytocin receptor antagonists have safety and efficacy comparable to that of nifedipine. However, they are costlier and not available in many regions.
- COX inhibitors may be used as tocolytic agents before 28 weeks of gestational age.
- Although magnesium sulfate has a tocolytic effect on the uterus, its use in preterm labor is confined to neuroprotection.
- The comparative effects for the baby of alternative drugs are unclear.

Based on the available studies and trials it was observed that nifedipine (calcium channel blocker) was the preferred drug for tocolysis in women at risk for preterm labor. WHO recommendations 2022 concluded that nifedipine was superior than other tocolytic agents in terms of risks versus benefits ratio, safety, efficacy, and availability. Although nitric oxide donors have comparative efficacy and safety profile to that of nifedipine, their exorbitant cost and nonavailability in all parts of the world render them less usable as compared to nifedipine.

American College of Obstetrics and Gynecology does not advocate any single agent as the first-line tocolytic agent although they do mention that nifedipine and indomethacin are the more popular tocolytic agents used.

Mayer et al. in their review mention that the choice of the tocolytic administered may be guided by the preexisting contraindications and allergies in the patient.

The COX inhibitors may be used for tocolytic therapy before 28 weeks of gestation. The WHO GDG group suggested that the use of COX inhibitors beyond this gestational age may be associated with premature closure of ductus arteriosus and oligohydramnios by affecting the renal function of the baby.

Lamont et al. in their review state that despite similar efficacy, beta mimetics and COX inhibitors are regarded as second-line tocolytic agents because of severe maternal and fetal adverse effects and concerns regarding the gestational age specific use. They also mention that nifedipine and atosiban have similar efficacy but safety profile is better with atosiban even though the cost is high.

Van Vliet et al. have also recommended the superiority of oxytocin receptor antagonists and calcium channel blockers over other tocolytic agents in terms of efficacy and side effect profile.

Xiong et al. in their meta-analysis comprising 44 randomized controlled trials and 6,939 patients have concluded that nifedipine was the most efficacious for delaying delivery followed by indomethacin.

Magnesium sulfate has long been used as a neuroprotective agent. However, its use as a tocolytic agent cannot be recommended because of lesser efficacy and more severe side effect profile as compared to the other tocolytic agents.

It should be noted that monotherapy is preferred to combination therapy as combination therapy does not have added advantage in terms of delaying preterm birth. Because of equivalent results it has been suggested that single agent should be used to minimize adverse effects while retaining efficacy.

The comparative effects for the baby of alternative drugs are unclear. Most drugs have been compared with beta-agonists. There are insufficient data on long-term follow-up for reliable conclusions about the effects on the baby for any of these tocolytic drugs *(Grade of recommendation-B).*

Calcium channel blockers were associated with less neonatal respiratory distress syndrome (RR 0.63; 95% CI 0.46–0.88), less necrotizing enterocolitis (RR 0.21; 95% CI 0.05–0.96) and less intraventricular hemorrhage (RR 0.59; 95% CI 0.36–0.98) than other tocolytic drugs. There was no clear difference between the treatment groups either in stillbirths (RR 3.00; 95% CI 0.13–71.07) or in neonatal deaths (RR 1.40; 95% CI 0.63–3.12).

Q4. What are the criteria for offering/not offering tocolysis?

Draft recommendations:

- The gestational age of the gravida should be between 24 and 33 weeks 6 days.
- Patient should be in suspected or diagnosed preterm labor.
- The administration of tocolytics should be offered together with the antenatal corticosteroid coverage and transfer to a better equipped center where the woman can have adequate delivery care and the preterm neonate can have adequate neonatal intensive care.
- Women should be informed regarding the possible risks and side effects of the tocolytic treatment being used. Contraindications of the proposed tocolytic agent should be ruled out before administration.
- Tocolysis should not be used in conditions where the continuation of pregnancy threatens the survival of the woman or the fetus (antepartum hemorrhage, chorioamnionitis) or is not beneficial (intrauterine death).

According to the American College of Obstetrics and Gynecology practice bulletin no 171, a gestational age >34 weeks, intrauterine fetal death, congenital anomaly of fetus that is not compatible with life, nonreassuring fetal heart, chorioamnionitis, eclampsia and vaginal bleeding are absolute contraindications for tocolytic therapy.

The ACOG also says that women who have premature contractions but do not have cervical changes should not be given tocolysis.

Hanley et al. in their review have also mentioned that the absolute and relative contraindications of the various tocolytic agents available should also be taken into consideration while planning the initiation of tocolysis.

NICE guidelines have also recommended that the woman should be assessed accurately and the diagnosis of preterm labor should be confirmed before offering tocolysis. The contraindications to continuation of pregnancy should also be evaluated.

Q5. What should maintenance tocolysis be used for?

Draft recommendations:

- Maintenance tocolysis can be considered after the acute regimen although no definite benefits were observed.
- Further research is recommended before maintenance tocolysis can be definitively advocated.
- Progesterone can be offered to maintain uterine quiescence after acute tocolysis.

Maintenance tocolysis may be defined as the continuation of the tocolytic drug beyond 48 hours or beyond the cessation of uterine contractions. WHO recommends that maintenance tocolysis may be considered although the benefits to the baby are yet to be established. ACOG advocates against the use of maintenance tocolysis as it does not culminate in improved neonatal outcomes.

Mayer et al. have mentioned in their review that progesterone may be used for the purpose of maintaining uterine quiescence although their use as tocolytic agents cannot be established.

Hanley et al. advocate against the usage of maintenance tocolysis as the risk versus benefit ratio is not supportive to the recommendation of its use.

In their meta-analysis of thirteen trials on maintenance tocolysis Breuking SH et al. have suggested the use of progesterone for maintenance after the acute tocolysis. Ferrari et al. advocate the use of progesterone for maintenance prior to 34 weeks of gestation as the effect is less pronounced after 34 weeks.

Hence, it can be concluded that although the use of tocolytics for maintenance tocolysis is still controversial, progesterone can be safely offered to women after acute tocolysis to maintain uterine quiescence.

Research gaps:

- Efficacy and effect of tocolysis in women with preterm premature rupture of membranes (PPROM).
- Effect of tocolytic treatment in women with multiple pregnancies.
- Long-term effects of tocolytics on both maternal and child health.

BIBLIOGRAPHY

1. American College of Obstetricians and Gynecologists' Committee on Practice Bulletins—Obstetrics. Practice Bulletin No. 171: Management of Preterm Labor. Obstet Gynecol. 2016;128(4):e155-64.
2. Breuking SH, De Ruigh AA, Hermans FJR, et al. Progestogen maintenance therapy for prolongation of pregnancy after an episode of preterm labour: A systematic review and meta-analysis. BJOG. 2023;130(11):1306-16.
3. Dagklis T, Akolekar R, Villalain C, et al. World Association of Perinatal Medicine (WAPM) and the Perinatal Medicine Foundation(PMF): Management of preterm labour: Clinical Guideline and Recommendation. EJOG. 2023;291:p196-205.
4. Ferrari F, Minozzi S, Basile L, et al. Progestogens for maintenance tocolysis in symptomatic women. A systematic review and meta-analysis. 2023 Feb 22; 18(2):e0277563.
5. Flenady V, Reinebrant HE, Liley HG, et al. Oxytocin receptor antagonists for inhibiting preterm labour. Cochrane Database Syst Rev. 2005;(3):CD004452.
6. Hanley M, Sayres L, Reiff ES, et al. Tocolysis: A Review of the Literature. Obstet Gynecol Surv. 2019;74(1):50-5.
7. Lamont RF, Jørgensen JS. Safety and efficacy of tocolytics for the treatment of spontaneous preterm labour. Curr Pharm Des. 2019;25(5):577-92.
8. Mayer C, Apodaca-Ramos I. Tocolysis.. In: StatPearls [Internet]. Treasure Island (FL): StatPearls Publishing; 2024.
9. Patel SS, Ludmir J. Drugs for the Treatment and Prevention of Preterm Labor. Clin Perinatol. 2019;46(2):159-172.
10. Pinson K, Gyamfi-Bannerman C. Antenatal steroids and tocolytics in pregnancy. Obstet Gynecol Clin North Am. 2023;50(1):109-19.
11. van Vliet EO, Boormans EM, de Lange TS, et al. Preterm labor: current pharmacotherapy options for tocolysis. Expert Opin Pharmacother. 2014;15(6): 787-97.
12. WHO. (2022). WHO recommendation on tocolytic therapy for improving preterm birth outcomes. Geneva: World Health Organization; 2022.
13. Wilson A, Hodgetts-Morton VA, Marson EJ, et al. Tocolytics for delaying preterm birth: a network meta-analysis (0924). Cochrane Database Syst Rev. 2022;8(8):CD014978.
14. Xiong Z, Pei S, Zhu Z. Four kinds of tocolytic therapy for preterm delivery: Systematic review and network meta-analysis. J Clin Pharm Ther. 2022;47(7): 1036-48.

7

CHAPTER

Role of Corticosteroids

Laxmi Shrikhande

Q1. Do antenatal corticosteroids reduce mortality and morbidity?

Draft recommendations: Antenatal corticosteroid therapy can adequately reduce the neonatal mortality and respiratory associated morbidity when given at the right gestational age between 24 and 34 weeks.

- Both betamethasone and dexamethasone are equally effective.
- Second dose of antenatal corticosteroid can be given after 7 days of the first course in special circumstances.

Do antenatal corticosteroids reduce mortality and morbidity?

In 1960, Graham Liggins in postmortem analyses, found that preterm lambs exposed to corticosteroids had structurally more mature lungs than expected and were also viable at an earlier gestational age and had less severe respiratory distress at birth.

1972 landmark study was a controlled study of antepartum glucocorticoid treatment for prevention of respiratory distress syndrome in premature infants.

Corticosteroids are administered to accelerate fetal lung maturity and reduce the risks of respiratory distress syndrome, intraventricular hemorrhage, and neonatal death.

Corticosteroids cause fetal lung maturity by two ways:

1. Stimulate surfactant release from type 2 pneumocytes
2. Direct action on maturing fetal lung structure.

Mechanism of action:

- Improving lung mechanics and gas exchange
- Increasing surfactant production
- Inducing production of surfactant proteins and enzymes
- Accelerate development of type 1 and 2 pneumocytes
- Inducing fetal lung antioxidant system
- Upregulating gene expression of epithelial Na channel.

At fetal gestational age (GA) of late preterm, the steroids benefit by increasing the expression of epithelial sodium channels (E Na Cs), alveoli convert active fluid secretion to fluid absorption and thus reduction in the fetal lung fluid and transient tachypnea of the newborn (TTN).

Q2. Can steroid be given more than once?

Dose:

- Betamethasone—2 doses 12 mg each IM 12 hours apart
- Dexamethasone—6 mg IM 4 doses 12 hours apart
- *Women between 24^{+0} and 33^{+6} weeks:* Maternal corticosteroids is offered.
- Repeat course of corticosteroids for women <34^{+0} weeks of pregnancy is considered when she had a course of corticosteroids >7 days ago (According to NICE, WHO) are a high risk of giving birth in next 48 hours.
- More than two courses of corticosteroids should not be used as they may have negative effect on the fetus.
- Comparative studies between betamethasone and dexamethasone show that both drugs are equally effective in preventing neonatal death and disability. However, dexamethasone has a faster onset and shorter duration of action, so is preferred in mothers with imminent delivery PPROM, diabetes COVID 19 infection, cardiovascular disease, and fetal growth restriction.

Antenatal corticosteroids can improve lung function only once adequate numbers of primitive alveoli and lamellar bodies appear in the saccular phase of lung development at around 25 weeks. Therefore, it is not of much benefit for RDS before 24 weeks (maternal fetal medicine unit network—RCT 2014). But steroid administration is controversial if the GA is between 34 and 36 weeks, as no sufficient data is available and no data is available about the long-term safety.

After one course of antenatal steroids, the maximum benefits are seen if the fetus is delivered 24 hours after and within 7 days of the last dose. Those who deliver within 24 hours of the last dose or even before the full course can be completed, do share some marginal benefits. It has also been shown that improved neonatal outcomes continue even beyond 7 days of the last dose and that the risk of RDS substantially decreases.

Single course of antenatal corticosteroids should be given to all women for an elective cesarean section planned prior to 38 weeks. There is still insufficient evidence on the long-term benefits and risks of multiple courses of antenatal corticosteroids. Repeat courses of antenatal corticosteroids will not help if mother does not deliver within 7 days. Since the benefit of a single course lasts beyond 7 days and given the evidence of adverse effects of multiple doses, it is strongly recommended that only a single course be used.

Q3. Which steroid is better?

Ans. Dexamethasone sodium phosphate is a more appropriate option and recommended over betamethasone because it is easily available, inexpensive, and heat stable. But dexamethasone has rapid onset of action and relatively shorter duration of action and therefore dosing frequency is more than that of betamethasone.

According to others, betamethasone seems to be a better choice than dexamethasone because:

- Betamethasone reduces neonatal mortality by a statistically significant degree.
- It decreases the incidence of periventricular leukomalacia whereas dexamethasone does not.
- Experimental animal data show enhancement of memory in mice with betamethasone and the use of dexamethasone decreased the memory level.

Both betamethasone and dexamethasone are identical in biological activity, both readily cross the placenta, both are devoid of mineralocorticoid activity, both cause weak immunosuppression and both drugs are extensively studied.

Q4. Are there any situations where steroid use can be restricted?

Antenatal corticosteroids should not be given when there is no substantial clinical concern for imminent preterm birth. Antenatal corticosteroids are also not recommended between 20 weeks 0 days and 23 weeks 6 days of gestation because there is a lack of data suggesting benefit.

Contraindications to the administration of antenatal corticosteroids include:

- Systemic maternal infection
- Maternal chorioamnionitis

Steroid injections during pregnancy can have side effects on both the mother and the fetus, including:

- *Fetal effects:*
    - *Low blood sugar:* Babies born after receiving steroids may have low blood sugar levels, which can be harmful if not treated.
    - *Reduced birth weight:* Babies exposed to steroids in the womb may have a lower birth weight.
    - *Mental health:* Some research suggests that babies born at full term who were given steroids between 22 and 37 weeks may have an impact on mental wellbeing later in life.
    - *Cleft lip and/or palate:* Some studies have linked corticosteroid use in early pregnancy to a higher chance of having a baby with a cleft lip and/or palate.
    - *Early-onset neonatal sepsis:* There is an increased risk of early-onset neonatal sepsis.
    - *Metabolic effects:* There may be increased amino acid concentration and fasting glucose levels.

- *Reduced fetal movements:* There may be reduced fetal body and breathing movements.
- *Reduced fetal heart rate variation:* There may be reduced fetal heart rate variation.
- *Reduced fetal intrauterine growth:* There may be reduced fetal intrauterine growth.

Guidelines:

- *The Society of Maternal and Fetal Medicine specialists:* Two doses of betamethasone for women 34–36 weeks with symptoms of preterm labor, cervical dilatation >3 cm, effective in 75%, and do not give tocolysis.
- *ACOG:* Dose as above, with imminent risk of preterm delivery within 7 days, chorioamnionitis is a contraindication and tocolysis should not be used. Single rescue dose if >2 weeks of last dose of steroid and GA <32–33 weeks with imminent delivery within 1 week.
- NIH—single dose at 24–34 weeks
- GOI NHM—single dose at 24–34 weeks
- *RCOG recommendations:*
    - Antenatal corticosteroids are associated with significant reduction in neonatal death, RDS, IVH, and safe for mother. It is not associated with any significant short-term maternal or fetal adverse effects.
    - They are most effective in reducing RDS in pregnancies that deliver 28–34 weeks.
    - For neonates delivered between 24 and 28 weeks, though the incidence of RDS is not much reduced, its severity is reduced and the incidence of IVH is also reduced.
    - Caution should be exercised when giving corticosteroids in women with systemic infections.
    - It should be given to all the women at risk of preterm birth up to 36 weeks.
- According to some studies, do not administer corticosteroid for women undergoing CS at >37 weeks. For vaginal delivery >34 weeks, do not administer steroid. TTN is less common in vaginal delivery.

BIBLIOGRAPHY

1. Ciapponi A, Klein K, Colaci D, et al. Dexamethasone versus betamethasone for preterm birth: a systematic review and network meta-analysis. Am J Obstet Gynecol MFM. 2021;3(3):100312.
2. Roberts D, Brown J, Medley N, et al. Antenatal corticosteroids for accelerating fetal lung maturation for women at risk of preterm birth. Cochrane Database Syst Rev. 2017;3(3):CD004454.
3. Roberts D, Dalziel S. Antenatal corticosteroids for accelerating fetal lung maturation for women at risk of preterm birth. Cochrane Database Syst Rev. 2006:(3):CD004454.

8

CHAPTER

Preterm Prelabor Rupture of Membranes—PPROM

Shanta Durge, Aaishwari Durge

DEFINITION

As per FIGO good practice recommendations preterm premature rupture of membranes (PPROM) is defined as rupture of membranes prior to 37 weeks of gestation and before the onset of labor or <259 days from the last menstrual period (LMP). This is similarly defined by the American College of Obstetrician and Gynecologist (ACOG), National Institute for Health and Care excellence (NICE), Royal Australian and New Zealand College of Obstetrician and Gynecologist (RANZCOG), and WHO guidelines.

Q1. How to diagnose PPROM?

Draft recommendations:

- Patient presenting with symptoms of PPROM like watery discharge per vaginum or the presence of pooling of amniotic fluid in the vagina as on per speculum examination.
- Additional laboratory tests can be considered to confirm the diagnosis. Amnisure seems to be promising simple and quick test with high sensitivity and specificity.

As per updated NICE guidelines: After a through history taking and sterile per speculum examination to take note of gush of watery fluid leaking through the cervix, should also look for cord prolapse, cervical status, and taking swabs should be taken for culture and sensitivity. Unless patient is in active labor do not perform per vaginum digital examination in view of the risk of introducing infection.

In equivocal cases, one can resort to further laboratory tests such as basic (nitrazine test, fern test, and fetal fibronectin) and advanced tests (PAMG-1/Amnisure, IGFBP-1/Actinprom). If tests are positive, they should be considered in combination with clinical condition, her medical and obstetric history and gestational age before embarking treatment. A re-evaluation of the patient if findings are not correlating , should be considered.

If clinical examination and laboratory tests are negative, diagnosis of PPROM is negated and patient is advised to report back if she gets any symptoms of PPROM.

NICE guideline do not recommend nitrazine test due to its high false positivity.

As per FIGO good practice recommendations: In low resource setting basic tests can be performed and in high resource setting advanced tests can be considered. Amniocentesis with dye instillation is Gold standard test but it is not recommended due to its invasive nature. Ultrasonography has low predictive value but it can be used for baseline evaluation of fetal status, biophysical profile, fetal presentation, liquor amount, and as a prognostic marker in further assessments till delivery.

As per journal of gynecology and obstetrics of Canada, placental α-microglobulin-1 (PAMG -1)/Amnisure is based on the measurement of PAMG-1 in vaginal secretions which is a 34-kDa placental glycoprotein found abundantly in amniotic fluid (2,000–25,000 ng/mL) and vaginal secretions normal range is 0.05–0.2 ng/mL. Detectable range for positive testing is 5 ng/mL.

Amnisure, which detects PAMG-1 in cervical secretions, is a promising, simple, quick, and easy test with a high sensitivity and specificity (96% and 98.3%). Amnisure can be used from 15 to 42 weeks and is not affected by presence of semen, urine, blood, or vaginal infections.

Insulin like growth factor binding protein-1 (IGFBP-1)/Actimprom is another simple test with sensitivity of 95%, specificity 92.9%, and NPV of 95%. But cervical ripening, stretching of membranes, imminent preterm labor can raise levels and give false positivity. As per a meta-analysis by ref: *Montse palacio et al.* Amnisure is preferred over Actimprom.

In a study by reference: Sowmya Jain et.al. published in JOGI, β-hCG of >21.5 IU/mL in vaginal fluid can be a reliable marker in diagnosing PPROM, with accuracy of 96%, sensitivity of 100%, specificity of 92%, and NPV 100%.

In future MRI may play a role in diagnosis.

Differential diagnosis of PPROM: It includes UTI, rectovaginal/vesicovaginal fistulas, urinary incontinence, vaginitis, urogenital tract trauma/surgery, vaginal douches.

Q2. What is the medical management of PPROM?

Draft recommendations: Medical management in PPROM is individualized; based on patient's general condition, and access to maternal and neonatal care.

Patient with PPROM management needs to be individualized on many factors which may include her general condition, period of gestation and remoteness from term, fetal condition, access to obstetric ICU and NICU care.

Medial management includes:

- Antibiotics
- Corticosteroids
- Tocolysis

- Neuroprotection
- Fetal and maternal surveillance
- General care in cases of PPROM
- Special circumstances

Q3. What is the role of antibiotics in PPROM?

Draft recommendations:

- Oral erythromycin 250 mg four times a day for a maximum of 10 days or until the woman is in established labor (whichever is sooner).
- Intravenous ampicillin (2 g every 6 hours) and erythromycin (250 mg every 6 hours) for 48 hours, followed by oral amoxicillin (250 mg every 8 hours) and erythromycin base (333 mg every 8 hours) for 7 days.
- Roxithromycin (150 mg 12 hours apart for 7 days—per oral) + cefuroxime (IV 750 mg every 8th hourly for 48 hours followed by oral dosage of 500 mg 12 hours apart for 5 more days), as a prophylactic antibiotic in cases of PPROM, showed longer latency and less maternal and neonatal morbidity than the use of ampicillin.
- In patients with indications for intrapartum antibiotics prophylaxis (IAP) for intrapartum prevention of early onset neonatal group B streptococcal disease (EOGBS) —bacteriological testing for GBS carriage is not recommended for women with PPROM. IAP should be given once labor is confirmed or induced irrespective of GBS status in PPROM with viable fetus.

Use of broad-spectrum antibiotics play a vital role in prolonging latency of pregnancy, reducing the prematurity related morbidities along with significant reduction in maternal infections such as chorioamnionitis, neonatal infections, and need for oxygen therapy in neonates. Multiple regimens have been proposed in various studies showing effectiveness, with no clarity on superiority of A (updated 2022 NICE guidelines) and B (NICHD—MFMU trial).

Penicillins have remained a mainstay of antibiotics. An RCT conducted by ref: Sgayer Inshirah et al. demonstrates that since gram negative pathogens constitute to major etiology in PPROM and due to the possibility of emergence of resistance to ampicillin, use of roxithromycin and cefuroxime in comparison with ampicillin, showed lesser neonatal and fetal morbidities along with a longer latency, reduced intrauterine infection, intrapartum fever, need for postpartum antibiotics, endometritis, and wound infections. Few other studies have found azithromycin as an alternative in PPROM, an RCT by ref: Rupsa C Boelig et al. in adapt trial showed that azithromycin with daily dose of 500 mg for 8 days can be considered.

Co-amoxiclav alone is not recommended in PPROM due its association with increased risk of neonatal necrotizing enterocolitis.

Also clindamycin alone is not recommended by NICE guidelines due to its resistance noted in UK.

The Royal College of Obstetrician and Gynecologist (RCOG) recommends IAP for prevention of EOGBS with benzyl penicillin from onset of labor/induction regularly until delivery at a dosage of 3 g IV benzyl penicillin at labor onset/induction and then 1.5 g 4 hourly until delivery. For optimal effects the first dose is given at least 4 hours prior to delivery.

If allergic to penicillin:

- Severe allergy to penicillin (anaphylaxis, RDS, angioedema)- vancomycin should be used-1 g every 12 hours
- Moderate allergy - IV cephalosporin can be used- cefuroxime, 1.5 g loading dose followed by 750 mg every 8 hours.

Q4. What is the role of corticosteroids?

Draft recommendations:

- I—use of steroids for fetal maturity in cases before period of viability is not recommended.
- II—between 24^{+0} and 33^{+6} weeks-use of antenatal corticosteroids is recommended for all women with PPROM. Short-term tocolysis can be considered for steroid coverage.
- III—between 34^{+0} and 36^{+6}, use of antenatal steroids can be considered.
- IV—In cases of PPROM after initial steroid coverage and no delivery for 7 days, a single repeat course of antenatal corticosteroids can be administered if high risk for preterm birth within next 7 days.
- V—antenatal corticosteroids are indicated even in multiple pregnancies with PPROM and at risk of preterm birth without any alteration in dosage.
- VI—dosage—
  - Two doses of 12 mg intramuscular betamethasone 24 hours apart
  - Four doses of 6 mg intramuscular dexamethasone 12 hours apart

Discussion: As observed from guidelines by ACOG, FIGO, and RCOG, administration of antenatal corticosteroids is a standard of care in management of PPROM cases.

The RCOG guidelines recommends antenatal steroid for PPROM cases between 24^{+0} and 34^{+6} pregnancy of gestation (POG), and suggests consideration of antenatal corticosteroids between 34^{+0} and 35^{+6} weeks. Use of antenatal corticosteroid in late preterm (34^{+0}—36^{+6}) is studied by ref: Rekha Upadhya et al. in a retrospective study and suggests reduced neonatal morbidity, mechanical ventilation need, NICU admission, and hyperbilirubinemia needing phototherapy.

FIGO guidelines on antenatal corticosteroids recommended to offer steroids in PPROM even if the completion of course is doubtful as beneficial effects are observed within 4 hours from starting the course. Multiple pregnancy is not a contraindication to antenatal corticosteroids.

Maximum of 2 and not more than two courses of steroids can be given.

Betamethasone/dexamethasone, no superiority over one or other.

NICE and RCOG recommend the use of antenatal steroids in cases with diabetes mellitus with PPROM, with additional caution on glycemic control and insulin administration as needed.

In imminent delivery cases dexamethasone is preferred due to its shorter duration of action.

A meta-analysis by ref: McGoldrick Emma et al. which studied the maternal outcomes and suggested that there is little to no difference in risk of infections associated with antenatal corticosteroids administration and the benefits outweigh the risks.

Contraindication for steroid use—established chorioamnionitis is the only known contraindication.

For more information kindly refer to the Chapter 7 on Antenatal Corticosteroids by Dr Laxmi Shrikhande in this book.

Q5. What is the role of tocolysis?

Draft recommendations:

- I—short term tocolysis in cases of PPROM can be considered in cases <34 weeks for steroid coverage or for shifting of patient to higher center for better maternal/neonatal care.
- II—no tocolysis indicated for pregnancies >34 weeks gestation and for PPROM before period of viability.

The PPROM and use of tocolysis is controversial due to limited data. As per ACOG practice bulletin 217 and RCOG-GTG 73, the use of tocolytics can increase the latency to delivery but comes with a risk of higher chances of chorioamnionitis without much maternal/neonatal benefit. Hence, tocolysis should be cautiously used in setting of PPROM only to buy time for steroid coverage for fetal lung maturity or to shift mother with baby in-utero to higher center in situations with lack of facilities to handle prematurity and its consequences.

For more information on tocolysis, kindly refer to the Chapter 6 on Role of Tocolysis by Prof SP Jaiswar in this book.

Role of neuroprotection—$MgSO_4$

Draft recommendations: Neuroprotection with IV magnesium sulfate ($MgSO_4$) for women who have PPROM and are in established labor or having a planned preterm birth within 24 hours is recommended.

$MgSO_4$ acts as neuroprotectant against the fetal brain. The risk of cerebral palsy is inversely proportional to the period of gestation hence there is a need for neuroprotection. Apart from main mechanism (described in Chapter on $MgSO_4$) one more function of $MgSO_4$ is to increase levels of neuroprotective markers, brain derived neurotrophic factor (BDNF) which are produced by the brain after administration, preventing the possible CNS damage and permanent CNS abnormalities, Sastra Winata et al.

Guidelines:

- I—from 24^{+0} and 29^{+6} weeks of gestation-$MgSO_4$ is offered. FIGO, RCOG, GTG 73 recommendation.
- II—<32 weeks (ACOG)
- III—30^{+0} and 33^{+6} weeks. $MgSO_4$ can be considered-FIGO and RCOG GTG 73

Dosage—mechanism of action, side effects, monitoring, please refer to Chapter 5 on $MgSO_4$ by Dr Pikee Saxsena in this book.

Q6. What is the role of amnioinfusion in cases of PPROM?

Recommendations: Amnioinfusion in cases of PPROM is not routinely recommended.

As per RCOG GTG 73 guidelines; neonatal outcomes can be apparently improved temporarily by amnioinfusion such as prevention of umbilical cord compression, pulmonary hypoplasia, and the supportive evidence remains sparse.

As per a latest systematic review and meta-analysis of five observational studies and three RCTs by ref: Celik Ebru et al., showed no clear differences in latency to delivery and perinatal mortality rates in cases of PPROM treated with amnioinfusion verses standard care. This study includes only observational studies and sparse evidences supporting amnioinfusion, hence the findings need to be interpreted with caution as per the study.

Role of sealants: *Draft recommendation*—there is no evidence to suggest that the use of various sealants in PPROM are associated with reduction of PTB or improvement in maternal and neonatal outcome.

There is very small amount of published data addressing the risk and benefits of the various sealing procedures employed with the aim to restore a physical barrier against infection and encourage reaccumulation of amniotic fluid.

Research gap: There is a need of conducting prospective RCT for the commonly used sealants including amnio patch, gelatin sponge, collagen plugs, or fibrin sealants.

Q7. What is fetal and maternal surveillance?

Draft recommendations: Maternal surveillance is based on assessment of symptoms and signs such as malodorous discharge per vaginum, signs like tachycardia, hypotension, fever, abdominal pain, uterine tenderness, leukocytosis, rising CRP titers, and reduced appreciation of fetal movements.

Fetal surveillance includes nonstress test (NST) and biophysical profile, but the frequency of assessment depends on the clinical status, period of gestation, and associated complications.

Guidelines: NICE: Utility of NST is inconclusive, as assuring NST excludes fetal hypoxia/acidosis whereas an abnormal NST is always not suggestive of fetal hypoxia and acidosis. Fetal scalp electrode monitoring and fetal blood sampling is not recommended for PPROM <34 weeks.

Q8. What is the general care in cases of PPROM?

Draft recommendations: Outpatient care in a viable fetus with PPROM, is not recommended.

In patient treatment is recommended in imminent delivery cases.

ACOG—a comprehensive assessment of previable PPROM and the latency to delivery in the hospital, it may be considered for home care as per ACOG guideline with proper counseling and guidance for the woman for surveillance and emergency care.

As per a retrospective study by ref: Borgida, Adam F, et al. previable PPROM occurring as a complication of amniocentesis, performed for genetic purpose are managed expectantly as outpatient, after a thorough discussion with the patient and after giving optimum knowledge about what all precautions to be taken at home to the patient.

RCOG—GTG guideline 73,—the role of outpatient management is inconclusive and there is insufficient evidence to follow methods of monitoring like ultrasonography to know AFI status and Doppler study and its interval.

In case of outpatient care, one has to consider several factors such as cost, safety, past obstetric history, support at home, and logistics with thorough counseling and after excluding the contraindications for expectant management.

From 24^{+0} to 28^{+0} weeks gestation delivery latency remains relatively constant at 8–10 days (median) and decreases to 5 days (median) at 31^{+0} weeks.

Q9. Explain PPROM and care in special circumstances?

- *PPROM with cervical cerclage in situ:* According ACOG practice bulletin 217 there is no sufficient and proven data to retain or remove the cervical cerclage in PPROM cases. In case it is retained, then antibiotics are considered for 7 days. There is a need for further study.
- *PPROM with herpes simplex:* ACOG guidelines states that herpes simplex with active lesions should be treated with acyclovir and patients with active genital lesions should be delivered by cesarean section.

- *PPROM and HIV:* In those cases of very early PPROM with HIV with low viral load and who are on ART treatment, can be considered for expectant management with strict monitoring.

Q10. What are complications of PPROM?

Fetal complications:

- *Prematurity:* The dreaded consequence of PPROM is preterm birth with its inherent perinatal morbidity and mortality and in 70-75% of cases giving rise to neurodevelopmental disability. India recorded the highest number of preterm births, at 3 million in 2018 as mentioned by FIGO in good practice guideline recommendations. About 50 % of women with PPROM deliver within one week of membrane rupture and there is inverse proportion between gestational age at PPROM and latency period. Clinically, evident intra-amniotic infection occurs in 15-35% according to ACOG.
- Perinatal morbidity due to pneumonia and neonatal sepsis
- Perinatal mortality
- Respiratory distress syndrome in infant (most common)
- Intraventricular hemorrhage.
- Neurodevelopmental impairment and increased risk of fetal white matter damage.
- Fetal lung hypoplasia—it is the lethal complication of PPROM in <24 weeks gestation secondary to oligohydramnios and impairment in fetal lungs canalicular development phase. Its incidence is 2-20% overall with perinatal mortality of 90%. The incidence is 50% at 19 weeks and 1% at 31.1 weeks as mentioned in book practical obstetrics problems by Ian Donald.
- Skeletal deformities—1.5-38%—but many of these resolve with postnatal growth and physical therapy.
- NICU admissions, prolonged stay in NICU.
  - Assisted ventilation
  - Increased cost of therapy
- *Obstetrical complications:*
  - Cord compression
  - Cord prolapse
  - Retained placenta
  - Placental abruption—2-5%
- *Maternal complications:*
  - Chorioamnionitis in15-25% of women and endometritis
  - PPH
  - Risks of preterm cesarean section and its complication

Q11. What are the indications for delivery?

The indications include:

- Nonreassuring fetal status
- Acute chorioamnionitis—diagnosed with persistent fever, maternal tachycardia, malodourous vaginal discharge or frank pus leaking from external os, leukocytosis, increased inflammatory markers, uterine tenderness, and fetal tachycardia.
- Placental abruption and antepartum hemorrhage
- Major fetal anomalies
- Pregnancy crosses >35 weeks—immediate delivery versus expectant management should be a shared decision based on maternofetal situations, as expectant management comes with benefits as noted even in a RCT by Morris J M et al.—PPROMT trial.
- Cord prolapsed and cord compression
- Evidence of group B streptococcus infection (GBS). PPROM expectant management versus induction of:
  - Labor (PPROMEXIL) trial
- Active labor
- Monochorionic multiple pregnancy
- Hypertensive disorders

The decision for delivery should be made based on fetal status, the stability of mother, and gestational age.

Research gap:

- Further studies are required to determine the antibiotic of choice and duration of treatment following PPROM based on Indian population prevalence of organisms and their sensitivity.
- Controlled trials are required to determine role of magnesium sulfate in PPROM when delivery is anticipated between 30^{+0} and 33^{+6} weeks of gestation. Comparative studies of a single bolus of magnesium sulfate versus longer intravenous infusion are required.
- Methods to monitor the fetus following PPROM require further studies.
- Further research is needed in the role of sealants to "repair" fetal membranes as well a role for amnioinfusion itself.
- More trials are needed to determine which groups of women with PPROM would not benefit from expectant management.

BIBLIOGRAPHY

1. ACOG Practice Bulletin Clinical Management Guidelines for Obstetrician-Gynecologists Number 217. [online] Available from https://www.acog.org/clinical/clinical-guidance/practice-bulletin [Last accessed November, 2024].
2. Baradwan S, AlSghan R, Sabban H, et al. Vaginal probiotics as an adjunct to antibiotic prophylaxis in the management of preterm premature rupture of

membranes: A systematic review and meta-analysis of randomized controlled trials. Eur J Obstet Gynecol Reprod Biol. 2023 Dec:291:112-119.

3. Borgida AF, Mills AA, Feldman DM, et al. 2000. Outcome of pregnancies complicated by ruptured membranes after genetic amniocentesis. Am J Obstet Gynecol. 2000;183(4):937-9.
4. Celik E, Yildiz AB, Guler Cekic S, et al. Amnioinfusion vs. standard management for the second trimester PPROM: a systematic review and meta-analysis of observational studies and RCTs. J Matern-Fetal Neonatal Med. 2023;36(2): 2230511.
5. College of Obstetricians and Gynecologists'Committee on Practice Bulletins—Obstetrics in collaboration with Robert Ehsanipoor,MD and Christian M. Pettker, MD. Prelabor Rupture of Membranes. [online] Available from http://unmfm.pbworks.com/w/file/fetch/140666496/Prelabor%20Rupture%20of%20Membranes_ACOG%20Practice%20Bulletin,%20Number%20217.pdf [Last accessed November, 2024].
6. Jain S, Jaiswar SP, Singh N, et al. Beta-HCG concentration in vaginal fluid: Used as a diagnostic biochemical marker for preterm premature rupture of membrane in suspected cases and its correlation with onset of labour. J Obstet Gynecol. 2020;70:283-8.
7. Kahvazi F, Rahimi K, Soufizadeh N, et al. The Effects of Vaginal Probiotic Administration on Perinatal Outcomes in Patients with Premature Preterm Rupture of Membrane. Arch Obstet Gynecol. 2022;3(2):59-63.
8. Mehndiratta M, Gupta B, Kar R, et al. 25-hydroxyvitamin Insufficiency in Pregnant Indian Women and the Development of Preterm Prelabour Rupture of Membranes. J Obstet Gynecol of India. 2021;71(6):649-50.
9. Moraes DV de, Junior E, Souza J, et al. "Does the use of probiotics in pregnant women with premature rupture of membranes improve the maternal and perinatal outcome? a systematic review". Brazilian J Sexual Transmit Dis. 2018; 30(3):102-6.
10. Nath B, Gaikwad H, Roy H, et al. Role of Vitamin C Supplementation in the Prevention of Premature Rupture of Membranes (PROM) and Preterm PROM: A Systematic Review and Meta-Analysis. Cureus. 2024;16(6):e62445.
11. Ronzoni S, Boucoiran I, Yudin MH, et el. Guideline No. 430: Diagnosis and management of preterm prelabour rupture of membranes. J Obstet Gynecol. 2022;44(11):1193-208.
12. Stock SJ, Thomson AJ, Papworth S, et al. Antenatal corticosteroids to reduce neonatal morbidity and mortality: Green-top Guideline No.74. BJOG: Int J Gynaecol Obstet. 2022;129(8):e35-e60.
13. Thom EA, Saade GR, Askie LM, et al. Prospective Meta-analysis for Pessary Trials Collaboration. Am J Perinatol. 2024;41(S 01):e2230-7.
14. Thomson AJ. Care of Women Presenting with Suspected Preterm Prelabour Rupture of Membranes from 24+0 Weeks of Gestation: Green-top Guideline No. 73. BJOG: Int J Gynaecol Obstet. 2019;126(9).
15. Ubom AE, Vatish M, Barnea ER, et al.; FIGO Childbirth and Postpartum Hemorrhage Committee. FIGO good practice recommendations for preterm labor and preterm prelabor rupture of membranes: prep-for-labor triage to minimize risks and maximize favorable outcomes. Int J Gynecol and Obstet. 2023;163:40-50.

16. Woodard PK, Wang Q, McKinstry RC, et al. Magnetic resonance imaging of the supra-cervical fetal membrane detects an increased risk of prelabor rupture of membranes. Front Endocrinol. 2022;13:1001538.
17. Xiong YQ, Tan J, Liu YM, et al. Cervical pessary for preventing preterm birth in singletons and twin pregnancies: an update systematic review and meta-analysis. J Maternal-Fetal & amp; Neonatal Medicine. 2020;35(1):100-9.
18. Zhuang Y, Li H, Na Q, et al. Prevention of preterm birth by cervical pessary combined with vaginal progesterone: a systematic review and meta-analysis with trial sequential analysis. Reprod Sci. 2023;30:93-110.

CHAPTER 9

Mode of Delivery in PPROM

Vidya Chaudhary, Sudha Sharma

Q1. How long can a case of PPROM be managed expectantly to improve the outcome?

Draft recommendations:

- Pregnancy, complicated by PPROM should be managed expectantly with maternal and fetal monitoring until 37^{+0} weeks who have no contraindication for continuation of pregnancy.
- Timing of birth should be decided on an individual basis with their preference and ongoing clinical assessment.

Management of PPROM depends on the gestational age at the time of leak. For late preterm (34–36 6/7 weeks) PPROM, either immediate delivery or expectant management up to 37 weeks is recommended and should be decided on an individual basis, level of NICU care, and clinical condition of patient (Grade A strong, moderate).

The Cochrane review (Bond DM et al., 2017) found no differences between early birth and expectant management in neonatal sepsis or infection. Early delivery increased the incidence of respiratory distress syndrome (RR 1.26; 95% CI 1.05–1.53), and an increased rate of cesarean section (RR 1.26; 95% CI 1.11–1.44). There were no differences in overall perinatal mortality or intrauterine deaths when comparing early delivery with expectant management. Early birth was associated with a higher rate of neonatal death (RR 2.55; 95% CI 1.17–5.56) and need for ventilation (RR 1.27; 95% CI 1.02–1.58).

The PPROM at previable age <24 weeks, termination of pregnancy should be offered with proper counseling regarding risks and benefits of expectant management versus immediate delivery by senior obstetrician with maternal-fetal medicine experts and neonatologist (ACOG Practice Bulletin No. 217, RCOG Green-top Guideline No. 73).

The PPROM after 24^{+0}–34^{+0} weeks should be offered expectant management with appropriate surveillance and counseling (Morris et al., 2016). 50% will go into labor within 24–48 hours. As with appropriate therapy and conservative management, approximately 50% of all remaining pregnancies deliver each subsequent week after PPROM, very few women remain pregnant >3–4 weeks after PPROM. Patients with PROM before 32w0d and imminent delivery are candidates for fetal neuroprotective treatment with magnesium sulfate (if no contraindications).

In certain circumstances, immediate delivery of the fetus with PPROM is indicated. These circumstances include chorioamnionitis, advanced labor, fetal distress, and placental abruption with nonreassuring fetal surveillance.

Reassuringly, a study by Noor E et al., 2023, suggests that both treatment options (IoL or EM) for patients with late PPROM do not affect short-term outcomes and long-term development of children until 10–12 years of age. This study provides the possibility of individualized healthcare and shared decision-making and helps clinicians to counsel parents not only on the perinatal outcomes, but also on the long-term developmental outcomes of their unborn child.

Recent randomized studies of preterm PROM (Pierre Delorme et al., 2021) show that EM until 37 weeks of gestation is associated with lower overall neonatal morbidity.

Research gap: More research is required in early PPROM group (<34 weeks) to determine benefit from expectant management.

Q2. When is the optimal timing for induction of labor in PPROM?

Draft recommendations:

- Late PPROM cases can be managed expectantly and those who have no indication for immediate delivery the optimal timing for induction of labor is ≥37 weeks.
- Early PPROM (<34 weeks) cases managed expectantly up to 34 weeks if condition permits, induce the labor between 34–36 weeks or earlier if lung maturity is documented

Pregnancies ≥34, expectant management is only recommended if gestational parameters are suboptimal; otherwise, expeditious delivery is preferred (Duff et al., 2019). Patients with PPROM should be admitted to hospital with periodic assessment for infection, placental abruption, umbilical cord compression, fetal well-being, and labor.

The decision-analytic model of PPROM at 34 weeks demonstrates that IOL at 35 weeks maximizes utility. This decision is most influenced by the risk of neonatal mortality at each gestational age. The optimal timing of delivery in PPROM is 35 weeks (Courtney Olson-Chen et al., 2016).

The most recent ACOG guidelines, updated October 2016, recommend induction of labor for women with ruptured membranes in the late preterm stages 34–36/6 days. This may present a challenge to widespread acceptance of expectant management for late PPROM.

A Cochrane review (Bond DM et al., 2017) are influenced by those trials assessing "late" PPROM (34^{+0}–36^{+6} weeks' gestation) such as the PPROMPT trial 2 and it is less clear whether expectant management to 37^{+0} weeks' gestation is appropriate for early PPROM.

Research gap: The variations in the guidelines reflect the heterogeneity of the literature contributing to the guidelines and challenges of diagnosing and managing cases of PPROM.

An improved international guideline may improve safety and outcomes in pregnant women with PPROM.

Q3. Which route of delivery is preferred for good maternal outcome in cases of PPROM—vaginal or cesarean?

Draft recommendations:

- Vaginal delivery should be the preferred mode of delivery for PPROM. It is associated with lesser maternal morbidity when compared to cesarean delivery.
- Plan for vaginal birth in the absence of maternal compromise or clinical indication for cesarean section.

The PPROM is a significant issue for obstetricians and an important cause of maternal and neonatal morbidity and somehow increased rate of cesarean section delivery.

Cesarean delivery is associated with increased maternal postpartum infections, admission to the Special Care Unit and even maternal death due to sepsis. The advantage of CS over vaginal delivery is expedited delivery of the distressed fetus but increases the maternal morbidity, so vaginal delivery is to be preferred to avoid postoperative morbidity.

NICE guidelines (2015) has mentioned that there are also difficulties associated with performing a cesarean section for a preterm birth, increased likelihood of the vertical uterine (classical) incision and its implications for future pregnancies.

A systematic review and meta-analysis (E. Demertzidou et al., International Society of Ultrasound in Obstetrics and Gynecology, 01 May, 2023) included 27 retrospective studies of 22,887 neonates) suggests that vaginal delivery in severe preterm birth is associated with an increased risk of neonatal and perinatal death in breech fetuses, while no significant association was observed for cephalic fetuses.

Research gap: Large multicentric randomized controlled studies are needed to definitively elucidate this dilemma.

Q4. Is there any difference in neonatal outcome in cases of PPROM being delivered by cesarean as compared to vaginal delivery?

Draft recommendations:

- For babies with cephalic presentation, cesarean section offers no specific advantage over vaginal delivery in the absence of any other complication.
- For breech deliveries cesarean section should be done unless delivery is imminent.

In a study (Jiang, Hai-Li et al.) 2,756 newborns were involved in the analysis. Among them, 1,166 newborns (42.31%) were delivered by CS and 1,590 newborns belonged to vaginal delivery (VD) group. After multivariable adjustment and stratification for gestational age, only pneumonia was significantly related with CS in 28–34 weeks group (OR, 0.34; 95% CI, 0.120–0.940; $p = 0.038$). This study concluded that the mode of delivery does not affect neonatal outcomes of pregnancies complicated with PPROM.

NICE guidelines (2015) mention that there are no known benefits or harms for the baby from caesarean birth. But cesarean section should be considered for women presenting in suspected, diagnosed, or established preterm labor between 26^{+0} and 36^{+6} weeks of pregnancy with breech presentation.

Queensland clinical guideline 2021 for preterm labor recommend vaginal birth unless there are specific contraindications to vaginal birth or maternal conditions necessitating cesarean section. For breech presentations the evidence regarding optimal mode of birth for preterm breech is conflicting and unclear due to a lack of high quality studies. The decisions should be based on individual circumstances and maternal preferences. Cesarean section is not generally recommended where vaginal birth is imminent.

Q.5. What is the cost effectiveness of expectant management versus induction of labor in cases of PPROM = or >34 weeks?

Draft recommendations: Expectant management is more cost effective as it improves neonatal outcome hence less admission to neonatal intensive care unit.

Jacqueline M Powell et al., 2022, demonstrated that expectant management of PPROM at 34 weeks has better outcomes than immediate induction of labor.

Recent randomized studies of preterm PROM (Pierre Delorme et al., 2021) show that expected management until 37 weeks of gestation is associated with lower overall morbidity and hence is cost effective.

Although there are no studies directly assessing the cost effectiveness of expectant management with induction, a study from PGIMER Chandigarh in 2005, mentions that the running cost of NICU care per patient per day was INR 5,450 (US$ 125). The average total cost of care for a baby <1,000 g was 1.68 lakh, between 1,000 and 1,250 g was 88,300 and between 1,250 and 1,500 was 41,700 and the family had to bear 25% of it.

According to an article by Neogi SB, the annual health system cost of operating SNCU at the district level is INR 6.3 million. The average cost of treatment per neonate is INR 4,581, while per bed-day treatment is INR 818, as reported from a study of four SNCUs.

In a study by *Karkambekar geeta et al., 2016,* the cost of NICU treatment in private facility was 90.7 US dollars (7,594 rupees).

So, given that there were no major statistically significant differences in outcome, induction of labor and early delivery definitely has a risk of being less cost effective.

Research gap: More health and cost effectiveness studies are required in this aspect of the problem.

Q6. Is it better to assess fetal lung maturity in cases of PPROM at 32–33 6/7 weeks and deliver or to manage expectantly till 34 weeks?

Draft recommendations: It is better to assess fetal lung maturity if facility is available in case of PPROM at 32–33 6/7 weeks and deliver accordingly.

The absence of fetal pulmonary maturity in patients with preterm premature rupture of the membranes (PPROM) is considered an indication for expectant management. In cases of PPROM <34 weeks, it is better to assess fetal lung maturity [fluorescent polarization test (surfactant/albumin), LS ratio, lamellar body count, presence of phosphatidyl glycerol].

Once the lung is mature then there is no benefit of expectant management rather there is still risks of infection, so the risks of infection outweigh the potential benefits of expectant management.

In patients with PPROM, delivery after confirmation of FLM at 32–33 6/7 weeks compared with expectant management until 34 weeks may prevent maternal infection without increasing neonatal morbidity (Akila et al.).

Sample for amniotic fluid can be obtained through per vaginal speculum and it is better than the amniocentesis for amniotic fluid as it has risks of procedure itself.

Research gap: There are very few studies done in this field, larger multicentric studies are required to assess the fetal lung maturity in cases of PPROM at 32–34 6/7 weeks and their impact on neonatal outcome.

BIBLIOGRAPHY

1. Bond DM, Middleton P, Levett KM, et al. Planned early birth versus expectant management for women with preterm prelabour rupture of membranes prior to 37 weeks gestation for improving pregnancy outcome. Cochrane Database of Syst Rev. 2017;3(3):CD004735.
2. Delorme P, Lorthe E, Sibiude J, et al. Preterm and term prelabour rupture of membranes. A review of timing and methods of labour induction. Best Pract Res Clin Obstet Gynaecol. 2021;77:27-41.
3. Duff PM. Preterm Prelabor Rupture of Membranes: Management. Am J Obstet Gynecol. 2023;228(3):326.e1-326.e13.
4. Hai-Li J, Chang L, Xiao-Xin W, et al. Cesarean section does not affect neonatal outcomes of pregnancies complicated with preterm premature rupture of membranes. Chin Med J. 2020;133(1):25-32.
5. Kayiga H, Lester H, Amuge PM, et al. Impact of mode of delivery on pregnancy outcomes in women with premature rupture of membranes after 28 weeks

of gestation in a low-resource setting. A prospective cohort study. Plos One. 2018;13(1):e0190388.

6. Melamed N, Berghella V, Ananth CV, et al. Optimal timing of labor induction after prelabor rupture of membranes at term: a secondary analysis of the TERMPROM study. Am J Obstet Gynecol. 2023;228(3):326e1-e13.
7. NICE guideline [NG25]Published: 20 November 2015 Last updated: 10 June 2022.
8. Powell JM, Clark, Jamie O. Lo, et al. Expectant management of preterm premature rupture of membranes at 34 weeks. A cost effectiveness analysis. J Matern Fetal Neonatal Med. 2022;35(25):9136-44.
9. Prelabor Rupture of Membranes. ACOG Practice Bulletin, Number 217. Obstet Gynecol. 2020;135(3):e80-e97.
10. Queensland guidelines: Preterm labour and birth. [online] Available from www.health.qld.gov.au/qcg [last accessed November, 2024].
11. ROCG. Green-top Guideline No. 73, Care of Women Presenting with Suspected Preterm Prelabour Rupture of Membranes from 24+0 Weeks of Gestation. [online] Available from https://www.rcog.org.uk/guidance/browse-all-guidance/green-top-guidelines/care-of-women-presenting-with-suspected-preterm-prelabour-rupture-of-membranes-from-24plus0-weeks-of-gestation-green-top-guideline-no-73/ [Last accessed November, 2024].
12. Ronzoni S, Boucoiran I, Yudin MH, et al. Guideline No. 430: Diagnosis and management of preterm prelabour rupture of membranes. J Obstet Gynecol Canada. 2022;44(11):1193-208.
13. Simons NE, de Ruigh AE, van't Hooft J, et al. Childhood outcomes after induction of labor or expectant management for preterm prelabor rupture of membranes. A 10-year follow-up of the PPROMEXIL trials. Am J Obstet Gynecol. 2023;588:e1-13.
14. Stancu SMK, Ash LK, Smeding C, et al. Predictors of Caesarean Delivery in Preterm Premature Rupture of Membranes. Open Access Maced J Med Sci. 2019;15(7):1124-8.

10

CHAPTER

Preterm Labor

Rajshree Katke, Anumeha Prasad

Q1. What are the maternal morbidities associated with preterm delivery?

Draft recommendations: Preterm delivery is associated with multiple maternal complications ranging from bleeding, infection, intensive care unit (ICU) admission, postpartum depression, difficulty in breastfeeding, and bonding with the baby.

There is increased risk of bleeding, infection, and ICU admission, especially in early preterm pregnancies due to T- or J-shaped uterine incision. Preterm delivery can be a stressful period for the mother who may experience anxiety, inadequate bonding with the child, difficulty in breastfeeding, postpartum depression, and post-traumatic stress disorder (PTSD). There may be an increased financial burden on the family due to neonatal intensive care unit(NICU) admission, long-term complications such as cerebral palsy. The parents may to be out of work for a prolonged period due to increased demand for care of the premature baby. The next pregnancy usually requires close monitoring due to increased risks of preterm delivery. Patients may need a repeat cesarean section in the next pregnancy due to weak uterine scar.

Research gap: Further research is required on the emotional aspects of preterm delivery including postpartum depression, bonding with the child, and traumatic disorders PTSD.

Q2. What are the potential long-term and short-term complications of preterm labor on babies?

Draft recommendations: Premature babies may have respiratory, neurological, cardiovascular, gastrointestinal, hepatic, and immune challenges.

Due to the different under developed organs premature babies can have multiple complications such as:
- Low birth weight and its implications.
- Respiratory distress syndrome due to immaturity of the lung and surfactant deficiency.
- Impaired immune system leading to neonatal sepsis.
- Neonatal jaundice due to immaturity of the infant's liver to process bilirubin. This can affect almost 80% of the infants.

- Anemia as result of increased breakdown of red blood cells.
- Necrotizing enterocolitis due to underdeveloped intestine which is more prone to infection, inflammation, and insults or injury.
- Intraventricular hemorrhage and other long-term problems such as cerebral palsy, epilepsy, and hearing loss.
- Retinopathy of prematurity and visual impairment.
- Developmental milestones may be delayed.
- There is increased likelihood of autism.
- Premature infants may have long-term health conditions. These include childhood obesity, asthma, and increased susceptibility to allergies

Q3. What postnatal care interventions are most effective in reducing neonatal morbidities including Kangaroo mother care (KMC)?

Draft recommendations: Timely interventions in the form of immediate NICU care or KMC including exclusive breastfeeding and enteral caffeine therapy in appropriately selected cases can effectively reduce neonatal morbidities.

- *Kangaroo mother care (KMC):* The World Health Organization (WHO) endorses the use of this method. KMC involves placing the preterm baby securely on the mother's chest with a binder to ensure an open airway. The birth partner can also provide the care the mother's absence. This method is suitable for babies who are as young as 26 weeks and weigh 600 g. This simple practice can be started in the hospital setting and continued even at home. There is evidence that suggests that KMC also increases the sleep time, tends to increase the duration of breastfeeding, results in higher milk volumes, and has positive effects on mother-to-child bonding.
- *Exclusive breastfeeding for 6 months:* WHO recommends that this practice fulfils the nutritional needs of preterm babies, in addition to offering other well-known benefits.
- Enteral caffeine therapy can be used to manage apnea of prematurity (AOP). The role of caffeine is to act as a central respiratory stimulant. This can improve breathing patterns of the premature babies and reduces morbidity related to apnea. This can be given orally or via a nasogastric tube.
- *Iron supplementation:* As human milk is deficient in iron, additional iron supplements are required for preterm babies.
- World Health Organization recommends supplementation with zinc and vitamin A in preterm infants can be considered.

Care of complications in preterm: The exact model of care for preterm infants varies globally depending on local protocols and available resources.

Neonatal intensive care unit (NICU) admission is not required in every case. The level of support varies and depends upon the gestational age, birth weight, and the presence of complications such as respiratory distress syndrome (RDS), tachypnea of prematurity, or neonatal sepsis.

The 2023 framework established by the British Association of Perinatal Medicine has a guideline that provides recommendations on the level of care that neonates might require based on their gestational age and birth weight.

Initial special care is provided to infants born between 32^{+0} and 33^{+6} weeks of gestation with any birth weight, initial care typically involves for babies born between 34^{+0} and 35^{+6} weeks with a birth weight below 1,600 g, initial care usually involves special care. If the birth weight is above 1,600 g, the initial care may consist of either special care or neonatal transitional care.

For babies born between 36^{+0} and 36^{+6} weeks of gestation with any birth weight, the initial care could involve either special care or neonatal transitional care. If the birth weight falls between 1,600 g and 2,000 g, neonatal transitional care is often recommended. If the birth weight is above 2,000 g, normal care with enhanced monitoring is typically provided.

Outline on management of RDS in preterm babies:

- The administration of steroid injections such as betamethasone or dexamethasone to pregnant women experiencing threatened preterm labor significantly decreases the occurrence and severity of RDS in premature infants. The Indian Academy of Pediatrics (IAP) endorses the importance of ensuring access to antenatal care and timely steroid administration for such patients.
- Diagnosis of RDS is based on a combination of factors that includes medical history, and clinical examination, and is confirmed by chest X-ray findings.
- Surfactant therapy should be initiated early in preterm infants born with signs of RDS preferably within 2 hours to reduce the need for mechanical ventilation. Additionally, WHO recommends early use of surfactants in preterm infants that require mechanical ventilation.
- Continuous positive airway pressure (CPAP) is recommended by WHO in preterm infants with clinical signs of respiratory distress syndrome. Early use of continuous positive airway pressure reduces the need for intubation and mechanical ventilation.
- Various methods, including radiant warmers and thermal mattresses, are effective in maintaining body temperatures in preterm infants to prevent hypothermia and its complications.
- The Indian Academy of Pediatrics (IAP) recommends incorporating enteral caffeine therapy into the management.

- The Indian Academy of Pediatrics provides specific recommendations for monitoring and managing metabolic imbalances that includes preventing hypoglycemia, hypocalcemia, and correction of hematocrit.
- Early initiation of enteral nutrition, preferably human milk, supports gut development and reduces the risk of necrotizing enterocolitis in preterm infants.

Research gap: Ways and means of promoting exclusive breast feed still needs lot of research.

Q4. What are the intrapartum and postnatal care to reduce maternal morbidities in women with established preterm labor?

Draft recommendations: Vaginal delivery is the recommended option except in emergencies. Holistic support in the postnatal period to address modifiable risk factors and interventions to prevent future adverse outcomes in the physical, mental, emotional, and metabolic health of the mother.

As the primary method of childbirth, except in emergencies such as antepartum hemorrhage or cord prolapse. The current evidence highlights the benefits of vaginal delivery in reducing both short-term and long-term maternal health issues. Cesarean section increases the risk of a classical scar, leading to higher chances of bleeding, ICU admissions, and weak uterine scar, potentially resulting in scar dehiscence, or rupture in future pregnancies. A thorough discussion with expectant mothers to explain all potential complications before any intervention is crucial in navigating these complexities. Ensuring adequate pain relief during labor is essential for a comfortable and safe birthing experience. Augmentation of labor using oxytocin is not contraindicated.

In the postnatal phase, adhering to local protocols is essential. Placental histology can be sent as it commonly serves as a diagnostic tool across healthcare settings, helping identify underlying pathologies and guide management strategies in subsequent pregnancies.

Postnatal care also involves providing holistic support to address modifiable risk factors such as smoking and substance abuse. Such interventions are crucial for preventing adverse outcomes and promoting maternal well-being in future pregnancies.

In addition to physical health, addressing the emotional welfare of postpartum women is crucial. Debriefing sessions are of vital importance especially in cases of unfavorable neonatal outcomes. These measures help to alleviate anxiety, address postpartum depression, and mitigate post-traumatic stress disorder. In addition, referring to peer support group can beneficial too.

In summary, managing maternal morbidities effectively requires a comprehensive and empathetic approach to ensure the best outcomes for both mother and child.

Research gap: More surveys and interventions are required in optimizing maternal emotional and metabolic health.

BIBLIOGRAPHY

1. David AL, Soe A. Extreme prematurity and perinatal management. Obstet Gynaecol. 2018;20:101-17.
2. Early postnatal care of the moderate-late preterm infant: A framework for practice. London: RCPCH; Royal College of Paediatrics and Child Health; 2023.
3. National Institute for Health and Care Excellence (NICE). (2015). Preterm labour and birth. [online] Available from https://www.nice.org.uk/guidance/ng25 [Last accessed November, 2024].
4. Phillip RK, Ramaswamy VV, Chandel P. Preterm with Respiratory Distress. Indian Academy of Paediatrics (IAP) Standard treatment guidelines. Indian Academy of Paediatrics (IAP). [online] Available from https://www.iapindia.org/pdf/ch-062-stg-preterm-with-respiratory-distress.pdf 9789240058262 [Last accessed November, 2024].
5. World Health Organization (WHO). (2022). WHO recommendations for care of the preterm or low-birth-weight infant. [online] Available from https://www.who.int/publications/i/item/9789240058262 [Last accessed November, 2024].

CHAPTER 11

Neonatal and Infantile Outcomes

Sarita Agrawal, Phalguni Padhi

Q1. What are the neonatal risks in preterm babies?

Draft recommendations:

- Preterm birth is a major cause of neonatal mortality and morbidity.
- Preterm neonates can have short- and long-term complications thus all the preventive and early and late management strategies needs to be effectively implemented.
- Preterm neonates are also liable to have long term sequelae and may contribute to certain transgenerational consequences.
- Neonatal risks at birth such as respiratory distress syndrome (RDS), intraventricular hemorrhage (IVH), patent ductus arteriosus (PDA), sepsis after birth, and can have short-term complications such as periventricular leukomalacia (PVL), bronchopulmonary dysplasia (BPD), necrotizing enterocolitis (NEC), retinopathy of prematurity (ROP), anemia of prematurity (AOP), osteopenia of prematurity (OOP). So, preterm labor and deliveries should be managed in a properly equipped neonatal intensive care unit (NICU) with proper anticipatory care till discharge.

Preterm birth, defined as birth prior to 37 weeks gestation, affects 15 million newborns globally every year. It is the leading cause of under-5 child mortality worldwide and accounts for 1 million deaths annually. Increasing preterm births are associated with the greater availability of assisted reproductive technologies (ARTs).

Preterm birth is the single largest killer of children under-5 years of age, accounting for >1 in three of all neonatal deaths (first month of life), and neonatal conditions are the leading cause of lost human capital in the most recent estimates of the global burden of disease, unchanged since 1990 **(Table 1)**.

In India, an estimated 26 millions of children are born every year. As per Census 2011, the share of children (0–6 years) accounts 13% of the total population in the country.

The major cause of neonatal deaths as per Sample Registration System Report (2015–2017) are prematurity and low birth weight (46.1%). In 2019, India's neonatal mortality rate (NMR) was 22 per 1,000 live births and had one of the largest cohorts of preterm and low birth-weight neonates globally. One-quarter of global newborn deaths occur in the Indian subcontinent.

Major problems of preterm neonates is enumerated in **Table 2**.

TABLE 1: Neonatal disorders: the leading cause of burden of disease, 1990 and 2019.

Leading causes 1990 (% DALYs)	***Leading causes 2019 (% DALYs)***
1. Neonatal disorders (10.6)	1. Neonatal disorders (7.3)
2. Lower respiratory infections (8.7)	2. Ischemic heart disease (7.2)
3. Diarrheal diseases (7.3)	3. Stroke (5.7)
4. Ischemic heart disease (4.7)	4. Lower respiratory infections
5. Stroke (4.2)	5. Diarrheal diseases (3.2)
6. Congenital birth defects (3.2)	6. Chronic obstructive pulmonary disease (2.9)
7. Tuberculosis (3.1)	7. Road injuries (2.9)

(DALYs: disability adjusted life years)

TABLE 2: Major problems of preterm neonates.

System	***Short-term problems (within 7 days)***	***Short-term problems (within 28 days)***	***Long-term problems (within 1 year)***
Respiratory	• Respiratory distress syndrome (RDS) • Air leaks • Apnea of prematurity	Broncho-pulmonary dysplasia (BPD)	• Chronic lung disease • Reactive airway disease
Gastrointestinal, nutritional	• Feeding intolerance	• Necrotizing enterocolitis (NEC) • Growth failure	• Growth failure • Failure to thrive • Inguinal hernias
Immunologic, infection	• Immune deficiency • Perinatal infection • Nosocomial infection	Nosocomial infection	Respiratory syncytial virus
Central nervous system	Intraventricular hemorrhage (IVH)	Periventricular white matter disease	• Cerebral palsy • Neurodevelopmental • delay • Hearing loss
Ophthalmologic	–	Retinopathy of prematurity (ROP)	• Blindness, retinal • Detachment, • Myopia • Strabismus
Cardiovascular	Hypotension patent ductus arteriosus (PDA)	–	• Hypertension in adulthood • Pulmonary hypertension
Renal	• Water, electrolyte imbalance • Acid–base disturbances	Late hyponatremia of prematurity	• –

Contd...

Contd...

System	Short-term problems (within 7 days)	Short-term problems (within 28 days)	Long-term problems (within 1 year)
Hematologic	• Iatrogenic anemia • Frequent transfusions	Anemia of prematurity	–
Endocrine	• Transient hypothyroxinemia • Cortisol deficiency	Osteopenia of prematurity (OOP)	• Impaired glucose regulation • Increased insulin resistance

Q2. What is association of these risks with gestational age at birth?

Draft recommendations:

- The risk of adverse outcomes in preterm neonates increases with decreasing gestation age. Even delaying the delivery by a week significantly improves the short-term and long-term outcomes.
- Late preterm babies have significant complications in neonatal period, so continuing the pregnancy would be the optimal practice.
- As per a large study the survival at 28 weeks is nearly 50% and at 32 weeks is >85–90% in India. Common short-term morbidities of preterm neonates were sepsis, birth asphyxia, hyperbilirubinemia, and respiratory distress syndrome. Late and moderate preterm neonates were significantly more likely to receive resuscitation at birth, respiratory and nutritional support, and were less likely to be fed breast milk than term infants. Necrotizing enterocolitis is a common morbidity among preterm neonates.

The risk of adverse outcomes of preterm neonates declines with increasing gestational age. Birth weight, neonatal morbidities such as respiratory distress syndrome, sepsis, hypothermia, hypoglycemia, marital status, required resuscitation after delivery, no antenatal care, the plurality of pregnancy, sex of neonate, mode of delivery, noncephalic presentation, fifth minute APGAR score <7, maternal complication and did not receive kangaroo mother care (KMC) were factors influencing preterm survival.

Research gap: There is no large meta-analysis that will tell us about outcomes in neonatal and infantile period by gestation ages.

AIIMS Delhi Study: Outcome of extremely low birth weight (ELBW) infants from a birth cohort (2013–2018) at AIIMS Delhi was performed which gives us insight into outcome of these babies.

In this retrospective cohort study, data were collected for all ELBW (defined as birth weight <1,000 g) infants born at All India Institute of

Medical Sciences, New Delhi from 1st January 2013 to 30th September, 2018. Gestational age was calculated using the last menstrual period, the first-trimester ultrasonography, or by clinical gestational assessment within 72 hours by Expanded New Ballard scoring.

The study was designated to evaluate survival rates, short-term morbidities, and predictors of mortality in ELBW infants. Survival below 28 weeks was low with 45% survival below 28 weeks which improved to 80% for neonates born between 28 and 31 weeks. Overall survival of neonates <32 weeks was 62% in the study. Survival below 800 g was low with 15–45% survival (<500 g–15%;<800 g–45%) which improved to 89% for neonates with weigh between 900 and 1,000 g.

Nearly 40% of neonates in the study had morbidities with RDS (57%), BPD (38%), Culture positive sepsis (19%), IVH grade 3 (12%), and PVL (10%) being the common short-term morbidities.

EPIPAGE 2 study: In one of the largest studies done in France from 22 to 34 weeks gestation informs us about the outcomes in preterm neonates. A total of 0.7% of infants born before 24 weeks' gestation survived to discharge: 31.2% of those born at 24 weeks, 59.1% at 25 weeks, and 75.3% at 26 weeks. Survival rates were 93.6% at 27 through 31 weeks and 98.9% at 32 through 34 weeks. Infants discharged home without severe neonatal morbidity represented 0% at 23 weeks, 11.6% at 24 weeks, 30.0% at 25 weeks, 47.5% at 26 weeks, 81.3% at 27 through 31 weeks, and 96.8% at 32 through 34 weeks **(Table 3)**.

Late preterm neonates morbidity: A retrospective cohort study of LPIs (340/7–366/7 weeks gestation) born at a single tertiary care center, Kingston Health Sciences Centre, Kingston, ON, between April 2015 and February 2017.

TABLE 3: Death and survival as per gestation age.

Gestational age, week	*All infants (n = 6,696)*	*Deaths in NICU (n = 413)*	*Survival to discharge (n = 4,467) 95% CIs for the percentage of patients*
22–26	2,205	248 (23.5)	552 (52.4) (49.4–55.4)
27	478	62 (15.5)	329 (82.3) (78.5–86.0)
28	526	40 (8.8)	411 (89.9) (87.2–92.7)
29	561	17 (3.3)	486 (95.5) (93.7–97.3)
30	761	19 (2.8)	660 (96.9) (95.6–98.2)
31	931	18 (2.1)	836 (97.0) (95.8–98.1)
32	281	4 (1.5)	266 (98.2) (96.6–99.8)
33	363	2 (0.6)	351 (99.2) (98.2–100)
34	590	2 (0.3)	3 (0.5) 576 (99.1) (98.4–99.9)

Results: 286 LPI infants were born during the study period. Of those, 7 infants were excluded for antecedents of delivery not documented in the chart. Therefore, 279 participants were included in the study.

Neonatal outcomes by gestational age: Infants born at 340–6 weeks gestation were more likely to have received antenatal steroids (46.2%, $p < 0.001$), have lower birth weights (2,411 ± 525 g, $p = 0.001$), and have longer NICU admissions (14.4 ± 6.5 days, $p < 0.001$).

Infants born at 360–6 weeks gestation were significantly more likely to be small for gestational age (SGA) (18.3%, $p = 0.018$) and to have received delayed cord clamping (58.7%, $p = 0.017$).

Decreasing gestational age was associated with significantly increased risks of apnea of prematurity (50.4%, $p < 0.001$), hyperbilirubinemia (60.5%, $p < 0.001$), and the need for continuous positive airway pressure therapy (CPAP) (45.7%, $p < 0.001$).

Of the 126 infants born at 360–6 weeks, 64 infants (50.8%) required admission to the NICU.

Q3. What are the association of these risks with mode of delivery?

Draft recommendations: There is no increased risk for cephalic vaginal birth however in breech <32 weeks gestation CS should be the mode of delivery.

There is a Cochrane review on "Cesarean section versus vaginal delivery for preterm birth in singletons." Six studies (involving 122 women) but only four studies (involving only 116 women) contributed data to the analyses.

There was also no difference in neonatal seizures, hypoxic ischemic encephalopathy, or respiratory distress syndrome. There was also no significant difference between the two groups for abnormal follow-up in childhood or delivery <7 days after entry.

The authors' conclusion was there is not enough evidence to evaluate the use of a policy of planned immediate caesarean delivery for preterm babies. Further studies are needed in this area.

A systematic review and meta-analysis of preterm deliveries ≤32 weeks of gestation concluded that cesarean delivery should be the mode of delivery for preterm ≤32 weeks of gestation breech births due to the higher mortality in preterm infants born via vaginal delivery. There is no increased risk for cephalic deliveries.

Q4. What are the other factors affecting the neonatal and infantile outcome?

Draft recommendations: There is increased neonatal mortality associated with GA <26 weeks, severe birth asphyxia and sepsis.

These associated factors should be avoided in preterm deliveries by proper monitoring of pregnancy, antenatal steroids (ANS), magnesium sulfate, and asepsis routines.

AIIMS Delhi study sheds light on the other factors that affect the neonatal outcomes.

Extreme prematurity (<28 weeks) and its complications accounted for the most number of deaths (n = 47; 53%) followed by sepsis (n = 29; 33%). Median (IQR) age of death was 7.5 (3–49) days. Half of all deaths were within first 7 days of life, whereas death beyond neonatal period (>28 days) occurred in 31% (n = 27). Nearly one-tenth (n = 7) and one-fourth (n = 24) of all mortality happened within the first 24 and 72 hours of life, respectively.

On multivariate analysis, gestation <26 weeks (aOR: 4.1, 95% CI: 1.7, 9.6), severe birth asphyxia (5-minute Apgar score ≤3) (aOR: 4.9, 95% CI: 1.4, 17.6), RDS (aOR: 2.9, 95% CI: 1.4, 6.1), shock within 72 hours (aOR: 4.3, 95% CI: 2, 9.2), and sepsis (aOR: 3.0, 95% CI: 1.3, 7.2) were associated with mortality.

Q5. What are the Recommendations to reduce these risks?

Optimization of the preconception parameters along with good antenatal care early diagnosis of the risk factors and implementation of the preventive strategies intrapartum and postnatal could reduce these risks exponentially.

Interventions provided before PTB to reduce neonatal morbidity and mortality:

- Antenatal corticosteroid therapy is administered for women at risk of PTB from 24 to 34 weeks of gestation.
- Use of antenatal magnesium sulfate to prevent cerebral palsy.
- Antibiotics are recommended in all women with preterm prelabor rupture of membranes (PPROMs).
- In utero transfer to a center where NICU is equipped to handle preterm babies. In extremely preterm infants, birth in a nontertiary hospital and transfer within 48 hours are associated with poor outcomes when compared with birth in a tertiary setting.

Interventions in labor room/operation theater (LR/OT):

- Having a trained neonatal team available for resuscitation.
- Intrapartum fetal heart rate monitoring.
- Delivery by cesarean section if benefits outweigh the risks.
- Delayed cord clamping ideally for 60 seconds or more.

Interventions provided to the newborn to prevent deaths due to prematurity:

- *Thermal care immediately after birth: Thermal care for preterm newborns:* Thermal care can be effectively provided by *kangaroo mother care (KMC)* to clinically stable newborns weighing <2,000 g at birth.

  A "warmchain" to prevent hypothermia in the newborn child includes 10 steps: (1) warm delivery room; (2)immediate drying; (3) skin-to-skin contact; (4) breastfeeding; (5) postponing bathing and weighing;(6) appropriate clothing/bedding; (7) mother and baby together; (8) warm transportation; (9) warm resuscitation; and (10) raising training and awareness.

Other methods to maintain the baby's temperature include radiant heaters, polyurethane bags, cling films, thermal mattresses, incubators, and topical application of oil- or paraffin-based ointments.

- *Breastfeeding:* The slogan "breast is best" is not exaggerated. Breast milk not only has immediate benefits for the newborn, protecting against neonatal morbidity and mortality, but also has long-term advantages.
- *CPAP:* In view of the high proportion of deaths due to RDS, CPAP is recommended for the treatment of preterm newborns with this condition, and should be started as soon as possible.
- *Surfactant replacement therapy:* Surfactant therapy is recommended for preterm newborns with clinical and/or radiologically established RDS.
- *Oxygen therapy:* Preterm babies born at or before 32 weeks of gestation requiring ventilation should be given oxygen therapy with 30% oxygen or air (if blended oxygen is not available) and not 100% oxygen.
- Nursing care with adequate nurse patient ratio
- Prevention of infections
- Prophylactic caffeine

Interventions postdischarge from NICU:

- Family counseling
- Enrollment in high risk neurodevelopmental follow-up and early intervention program.
- Easy options for follow up under one roof: Pediatric neurology, ophthalmology, audiology and ENT, developmental pediatrician, occupational therapist, physiotherapist, etc.
- Immunizations

Small and vulnerable neonates "SVN"—a new concept: A new conceptual framework that brings preterm birth, SGA, and LBW together under the term "small vulnerable newborns" (SVN) in order to contribute to healthier and thriving women, newborns, children, adults, and societies by Lancet SVN series.

The relative neonatal mortality risk for each of the three SVN types compared with term nonSGA within each NMR band. The relative risk (RR) was highest for babies who were preterm, SGA or not, compared with term non-SGA. Risks associated with being both preterm and SGA were higher than for preterm alone in all mortality settings.

Research gap: Awareness regarding the understanding the healthcare providers regarding the link between optimization of the preconception parameters and the transgenerational effects of preterm birth and NCDs need to be included in the teaching curriculum.

BIBLIOGRAPHY

1. Alfirevic Z, Milan SJ, Livio S. Caesarean section versus vaginal delivery for preterm birth in singletons. Cochrane Database of Systematic Reviews. 2013;9:CD000078.
2. Del Río R, Thió M, Bosio M, et al. Prediction of mortality in premature neonates. An updated systematic review. An Pediatr. 2020;93:124-33.
3. GBD 2019 Diseases and Injuries Collaborators. Global burden of 369 diseases and injuries in 204 countries and territories, 1990-2019: a systematic analysis for the Global Burden of Disease Study. 2019.
4. Lorenzo M, Laupacis M, Hopman WM, et al. Morbidity in late preterm birth: A retrospective cohort study assessing the role of immaturity versus antecedent factors. Neonatology. 2021;118(3):317-24.
5. Ministry of Health & Family Welfare, Government of India. Child health. National Health Mission; 2022.
6. Ohuma E, Moller A-B, Bradley E (in press). National, regional, and worldwide estimates of preterm birth in 2020, with trends from 2010: a systematic analysis. Lancet. 2023;402(10409):1261-71.
7. Sahoo T, Anand P, Verma A, et al. Outcome of extremely low birth weight (ELBW) infants from a birth cohort (2013–2018) in a tertiary care unit in North India. J Perinatol. 2020;40:743-9.
8. Sharrow D, Hug L, You D, et al. Global, regional, and national trends in under-5 mortality between 1990 and 2019 with scenario-based projections until 2030: a systematic analysis by the UN Inter-agency Group for Child Mortality Estimation, Lancet Global Health. 2022;10(2):e195-e206
9. Unger V, Gasparics Á, Nagy Z, et al. Cesarean delivery is associated with lower neonatal mortality among breech pregnancies: a systematic review and meta-analysis of preterm deliveries ≤32 weeks of gestation. Am J Obstet Gynecol. 2024;S0002-9378(24)00683-5.
10. WHO. Born too soon: decade of action on preterm birth. [online] Available from https://www.who.int/publications/i/item/9789240073890 [Last accessed November, 2024].
11. World Health Organization, United Nations Children's Fund (UNICEF), United Nations Population Fund (in press). Together for change: for every pregnant woman, every new mother, every newborn. Geneva: World Health Organization; 2023.
12. You D, Hug L, Ejdemyr S, et al. Global, regional, and national levels and trends in under-5 mortality between 1990 and 2015, with scenario-based projections to 2030: a systematic analysis by the UN Inter-agency Group for Child Mortality Estimation. Lancet. 2015;386(10010):2275-86.